MODERN
AYURVEDA

MODERN AYURVEDA

RITUALS, RECIPES & REMEDIES FOR BALANCE

ALI CRAMER

Photography by Evi Abeler

ALTHEA
PRESS

Interior and Cover Designer: Amanda Kirk
Photo Art Director/Art Manager: Sarah Feinstein
Editor: Samantha Barbaro
Photography © 2019 Evi Abeler. Food styling by Albane Sharrard. Prop styling by Sara Feinstein.
Illustrations © 2019 Tom Bingham.
Author photo courtesy of © Denisse Monge.

ISBN: Print 978-1-64152-523-7 | eBook 978-1-64152-524-4

I dedicate this book to my biological and chosen family, my teachers, and my students. Thank you for inspiring me to Go. On. Duty. Namaste, Ali.

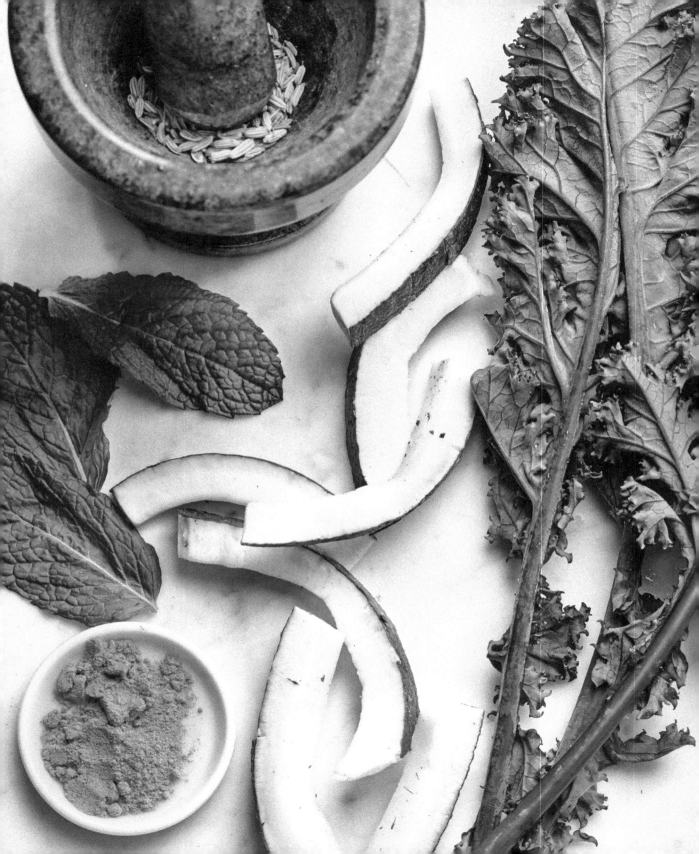

Contents

PART ONE
AYURVEDA TODAY

AYURVEDA IS GOING TO CHANGE YOUR LIFE. Yikes. Big statement on the very first page. You're right to be resistant, my Kapha friend, or skeptical, my Pitta friend, or confused, my Vata friend. You might have a combination or even all of those reactions. Those reactions could be ones that crop up a lot for you, so they may be familiar. Let's look at the unfamiliar words there: Kapha, Pitta, and Vata. Remember those words. That's your first assignment on the path to increased health and happiness the *Modern Ayurveda* way.

Chances are good that by now you have come across Ayurveda—it's increasingly referenced in wellness circles. Perhaps you've read an article somewhere, taken a workshop at your yoga center, or enjoyed one of the Ayurvedic turmeric lattes popping up at cafés. Maybe you've heard it's the sister science to yoga, or maybe you took an online quiz to find your *dosha* and your curiosity was piqued enough to pick up this book. Congratulations—you have a fantastic journey ahead of you! One that is filled with insight into self-care and aha moments that point the way to more understanding, healing, and compassion for ourselves and others.

Yes, I'll talk about what you should eat and drink and how much you should exercise. I'll also cover when and how long you should sleep, which hobbies and social habits suit you, and much more! Seem like unrelated topics? I challenge you to change your way of thinking, because Ayurveda is a system of holistic health, and it can inform every choice you make in your daily life. This book was created with a lot of love to help you understand the theories and principles that can guide and empower you in designing a unique lifestyle plan. But I'm getting ahead of myself here. Here's how it started for me.

My Path to Ayurveda

I was introduced to Ayurveda in 2003 in New York City, far from the beautiful shores of the birthplace of the practice in India. I was doing my yoga teacher training at Laughing Lotus yoga center, and we had a one-day introduction to Ayurveda. All of a sudden, through the lens of Ayurveda, the world made a lot more sense. I did my first Ayurvedic training that year, and went on to study with many great teachers. As my understanding grew, I began to incorporate the practices into my life and saw my life changing for the better. Eventually, it was time to start sharing what I'd learned; it had already influenced the way I structured my yoga classes and my work with private yoga clients. I started with short workshops and lectures, and in 2010, I moved on to teaching trainings. I'm now the director of the Ayurveda program at Laughing Lotus. In addition, I hold private Ayurvedic lifestyle counseling sessions, lead Ayurveda and yoga retreats, and guest teach both nationally and internationally.

Someone once said to me, "Wow, Ali, you really are a go-to Ayurveda resource in New York City! There aren't a lot of Ayurvedic practitioners here." To which I replied, "I guess that's true." And then I thought about it. *Of course* there weren't a lot of Ayurvedic practitioners in NYC. It's *difficult* to keep up an Ayurvedic lifestyle in New York City—and for that matter, with the demands of our modern lives and our modern technology, it's difficult no matter where you live. And yet, I have always believed there is a way to use Ayurvedic tools to bring more peace and health to your life as it is today. I believe that despite the non-negotiable aspects of modern life (demands of career, family, age, geographical location, or lifestyle choices), even small steps make a huge difference. My message to all of my students and clients has always been how easy it is to incorporate ancient Ayurvedic principles into our modern lives. I encourage a slow, loving approach, one that sets you up for success in your wellness goals.

This book provides Ayurvedic ways to support your healing as these teachings have been doing for thousands of years for so many throughout the world. We cover common imbalances, both physical and mental, and provide simple, practical solutions by using "prescriptions" that are easily filled at your local grocery store or online. My goal is to help you understand the basic theories and take suggested actions. I have found that the shifts you need to make for optimal health occur with more willingness when you understand the reasoning behind them. And what good is theory without practice? Use this book as a way to kickstart your next level of health—think of it as preventive care and solutions from Mother Nature with no dangerous or mysterious side effects. There are quick tips and longer cleansing plans, daily and seasonal practices, and healthy (yummy!) recipes.

Welcome to a lifelong path of shifting into harmony with the conditions of your life. Think of this book as a map to empower you with understanding and tools to take charge of your health and happiness! Let's get on with it! Harmony awaits.

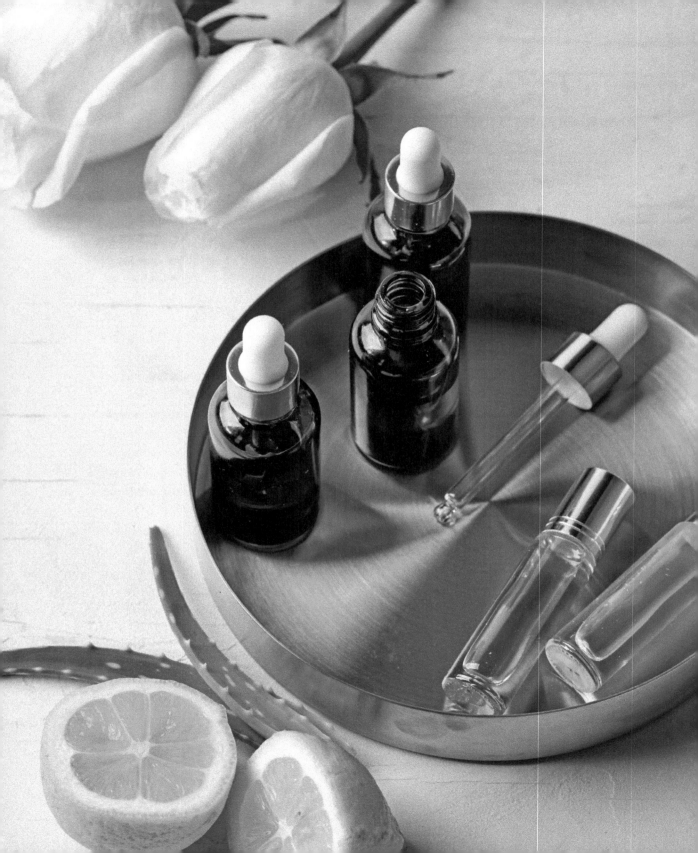

1

ESSENTIAL AYURVEDA

In this chapter, I cover the basic principles and
theories of Ayurveda. I believe the more thorough your
understanding of the reasons behind your actions,
the more likely you are to make lasting changes.

A Brief History of Ayurveda

Ayurveda is a Sanskrit word meaning "Science of Life." Sanskrit is an ancient and holy Indo-European language from India. Ayurveda came to be in the south of India. The oldest Ayurvedic texts cover recommendations for almost all areas of health care, from pediatrics and geriatrics to psychology, pre- and postnatal care, surgery, optometry, psychiatry, and plant remedies. It is a complete system based on the elements of nature and living a life in accordance with the natural rhythms of our world.

Optimal Health and Well-Being

The goals of Ayurveda are health and happiness in body and mind. Ancient texts tell us that if the body is "healthy" but the mind is sad, depressed, or angry, we still have healing to do. That's why we call it a system of (w)holistic health. We want to look at the whole picture of what health both looks like and feels like. A happy and peaceful mind should go along with a healthy body.

Achieving Balance

In modern society, so many of us struggle to find balance. You may work long hours and often take work home with you. You may have partners, children, family, or friends that you want to give time and attention to as well. Unfortunately, with such a full life, self-care can be the last priority. How many times have you found yourself in bed, phone in hand, sending that last e-mail or scrolling your Instagram feed? I've done it, you've probably done it, and there is that small voice inside of you saying, "Put the phone away and go to bed. You're exhausted." Ayurvedic theory tells you to listen to that voice, the one filled with common sense. And that's another thing I love about Ayurveda—it makes so much sense! Ayurvedic theory tells you that you keep all of the answers inside; you've just gotten out of the habit of listening. It's a skill. And one that can be practiced on a daily basis throughout your life.

What Is Modern Ayurveda?

So how do you bring Ayurveda into your life in a way that feels palatable, practical, and doable in the twenty-first century? Modern Ayurveda may look different from ancient Ayurveda because your lifestyle is different, but its basic wisdom is timeless! What makes Ayurveda relevant to modern times is understanding the theories behind the practices and using the tools within the parameters of our lives today. One of my teachers says that when something has been deemed worthy of passing down for a few thousand years, it's proved itself as containing truth. Ayurvedic wisdom has been proven throughout the ages to be a science that can relieve suffering, both physical and mental. So, how do you do it?

For starters, relax! You do not have to do a giant overhaul. Please know that small changes add up. One of my favorite quotes from one of my teachers is "Ayurveda meets you where you're at, but doesn't leave you where it found you." I love that! Let's dive into these theories to help you relearn how to align with your true nature. As a baby, you knew how to do it. When you were tired, you slept. When you were hungry or thirsty, you fussed until someone fed you or gave you something to drink. And for that matter, when you needed to poop or pee or burp or sneeze, you didn't hold it in or wait for an "appropriate" place or time. (Ayurveda talks about poop. We are going to talk about poop. Consider yourself warned.) I'm not suggesting you walk around peeing/pooping/sneezing/burping wherever and whenever you feel like it. Just remember that the body has its own intelligence and timetable, and doing your best to honor that makes everything run much more smoothly.

Ayurveda 101

Let's start with what I like to call Ayurveda 101. Here are my top three principles to keep in mind.

1. **Like increases like. Opposites balance.** This shows up in many ancient healing traditions. In traditional Chinese medicine, it's represented by yin and yang. In yoga, we refer to *stiram* and *sukham*, which means effort and ease. Ayurvedic theory backs up this relationship.

    Sometimes you are already doing this without even knowing it! I find this so often with my clients—the "bad" habits in their lives are actually serving a purpose and trying to balance them out in some way. Ayurveda merely recommends finding a healthier alternative. Are you too anxious (fast quality) to quit smoking or vaping? Try a meditation practice. Both smoking and meditation will quiet you down (slow quality). Both will take you away from what you're doing for a little while. Both will bring awareness around breath, and both will be calming for the nervous system. But over time, smoking will make you feel really bad. Over time, meditation will make you feel really good.

Or, are you so exhausted (heavy quality) that you start pounding double espressos (light quality) like it's your job? Get some peppermint essential oil, and put it on your nightstand. First thing in the morning, dab a couple drops on the soles of your feet and bring the bottle with you for a refresher when the caffeine craving hits. It's cheaper and way better for the adrenals.

TIP: If you get a caffeine withdrawal headache, put some peppermint oil on the occipital ridge—where the back of your hairline meets your neck. Reach back there; you'll feel two bumpy protrusions. Put one drop on each side.

2. **Ayurveda is not one size fits all.** We've all fallen prey to the latest fad or recommendation from a coworker or family member who feels "amazing" after eliminating or adding a certain food or supplement or trying a new fitness trend or body treatment. And yet, when you do the same, you feel terrible. Ayurvedic principles say try a different way—curate a health plan that is unique to your needs; unique to your constitution.

3. **Ayurveda is not a quick fix.** Yes, in the flare-up of a headache there are Ayurvedic tools that will help relieve the pain. But let's also look at the bigger picture. What if you could do things on a daily basis for a year or so that would help ensure the headaches are occurring far less often and with less intensity? What if you continue said things for a long enough time that one day you realize you actually haven't had a headache in God-knows-how-long? I can't give you any guarantees or tell you how long it will take, but you can take consistent small steps to ensure you are doing all you can to stay healthy. What an empowering way of living!

Living by the Natural Rhythms of Life

Keep these three principles in mind, and let's take a closer look at the world we live in. Here's another Sanskrit word to learn: *Panchamahabhutas*. It refers to the five great elements of our world: earth, water, fire, wind, and space. On their own or in combination, they make up everything you know: the seasons, time of day, time of life, your body, the food you eat, the thoughts you think. Everything! The entire Ayurvedic system revolves around working with these elements and finding a balance among them. When you have the proper ratios of each present, you feel balanced. When the ratios are off, you can fall into dis-ease.

Seasons

Take the seasons, for instance. Ayurveda separates the calendar into three distinct seasons. Each is associated with two elements. Late winter into spring is associated with earth and water; it's called Kapha season. If we put earth and water together, we get mud. Kapha season is muddy. And I often find this is the time of year when my clients and I can feel "muddy." Maybe we have gained a little weight, have been spending too much time indoors, burrowing under blankets, and we start to feel a little sluggish, or even mildly depressed. Seasonal affective disorder is real! One of my clients, Trisha, came to me in the winter complaining of exactly these symptoms. I listened to her, looked her over, and asked her a bunch of Ayurvedic diagnostic questions. One of many recommendations I gave her was to start taking vitamin D. I always like to be as cautious as possible with herbs and supplements, so I advised her to visit her regular Western general practitioner for a full physical and suggested she start taking 1,000 IU of vitamin D a day. The following week she went to her doctor, and sure enough, she had a major vitamin D deficiency. He backed me up in supplementing with vitamin D and approved of all the dietary shifts and other recommendations. That's another way that Ayurveda can be modernized; it can partner with Western medicine to create optimal health.

> **TIP:** Always get regular physicals, dentist appointments, and gynecological care. I never advise anyone to go off or on a medication.

Back to the seasons. Next up is late spring into summer, called Pitta season. It's the hottest time of the year, associated with the elements of water and fire. For the Northern Hemisphere, think of the warmth of June and July bookended on either side by the rains of May and humidity of August. Initially, after the long, cold winter, that heat feels so good. By August, it has become a bit much, and you can find yourself feeling overheated, itchy, irritable, or a combination of all three.

Happily, our next season is a bit lighter and cooler. The third season is autumn into early winter, or what we call in Ayurveda Vata season. That first chilly evening feels refreshing, even exciting, but by December you can feel a bit dried out and exhausted.

Are you seeing the pattern here? Nature is trying to balance itself out. Each season is rebounding from the last. Vata season is cold and light and dry, Kapha season is cold, sure, but also heavy and wet. Pitta season is wet, sure, but also hot and light, which goes back into Vata season, which is light, sure, but also cold and dry, and so on. You see the pattern. This pattern plays out in time of day as well.

Ayurvedic Seasons

Kapha Season	Pitta Season	Vata Season
Winter into early spring	Spring into early summer	Autumn into early winter

So far so good? Great; let's move on to time of day.

Day and Night

Have you ever woken up around 4:30 a.m. when you didn't have to? No work that day, no appointments or commitments. And you feel awake, clear, ready to go, but somewhere in your head you're like, "Well, I don't have to be up now," so you turn over and manage to fall back asleep. You wake up again at 8:00 a.m., and instead of feeling better, you somehow feel worse? You're now sluggish and out of it, so you hit the kitchen to make a strong coffee for yourself to clear your head. This is Ayurveda at work! Let me explain.

Ayurveda divides the day into four-hour increments and assigns one of the previously mentioned "seasons" to them. Each season, as we know, has an energetic quality to it. Here's a quick recap:

- **Kapha season** is cold and heavy and wet and slow
- **Pitta season** is hot and light and wet and fast
- **Vata season** is cold and light and dry and fast

Our Inner Rhythms

Let's now place these energies into your daily timetable. Again, this will make so much sense when you think about it!

Vata time of day is 2:00 to 6:00 a.m. and 2:00 to 6:00 p.m. No wonder you woke up at 4:30 a.m. and felt alert. And think about that midafternoon time. It's that time of day when you feel a little restless, maybe you get up from your desk and start poking around for a little snack, or realize you need to stretch your legs and drink some water (great) or an energy drink or hit the candy jar (not so great, and I'll get into why in a bit). Think about how many cultures take a pause around this time. There are many places in the world where teatime happens around 3:00 p.m. In some of the hotter countries, it's the time for siesta. It's like we need a reset, a little shift in our day before it ends.

Let's go back to the early rising example. You felt ready to go at 4:30 a.m., but then when you woke up at 8:00 a.m., you felt draggy. One could even say muddy. There's your clue. From 6:00 to 10:00 a.m. and 6:00 to 10:00 p.m. is Kapha time. Most of the world wakes up around then, and most of the world reaches for caffeine in some form at that time. Ayurveda in action! Kapha is wet; coffee is drying. Kapha is slow; caffeine speeds things up. Sometimes, for clients who struggle with waking up in the morning, I might recommend they get up earlier to bypass some of that heavy Kapha energy. In the evening, though, we want to use some of that slowness, even the heaviness. Have you noticed that if you go to sleep around 10:00 or 10:30 p.m., you sleep more deeply and easily? In Western culture it's called the circadian rhythm. Ayurveda calls it living in harmony.

Same-same. Four thousand years ago, when it was dark, you went to sleep. When it started to get light outside, you woke up. There was no YouTube, Hulu, or Netflix. Let's take this as wisdom, that stretching our workday or leisure time past midnight might not be the best thing for our health.

This is because 10:00 a.m. to 2:00 p.m. and 10:00 p.m. to 2:00 a.m. is governed by Pitta time. The sun is the strongest, and our digestion is the strongest. The fire needs to be fed! In Ayurvedic theory, for Pitta time, we should use some of that Pitta energy and be super productive, and then make sure we stop to have a good lunch, as this is when our digestive fire is the strongest. This can backfire on us if we stay awake into Pitta nighttime. How many of us have had a good dinner, stayed up late even though we were a bit tired, and somewhere around 11:30 p.m. or midnight wandered into the kitchen with the munchies? And it's not kale salad we want at midnight. It's one or more of the following: crunchy, salty, creamy, sweet. I get it! I've been there! I might go there again! But isn't it a relief, somehow, to know why? And that we could take a simple side step and avoid it? Go. To. Sleep!

Aging

Ayurveda also says that your age can affect you. From babyhood to around the teens, we have more Kapha energy. Think of how easily children get colds and runny noses; it's the cold and wet qualities at work. From our teens to around our 50s, we have more Pitta. You need some of that fire to venture out into the world, to learn your skills and succeed in your jobs before you arrive in older age. If it's summer and noon, and you are in your mid-30s, there is a *lot* of that Pitta energy in the world around you. If you put that together with suboptimal lifestyle choices, that fire can rage out of control! The next phase of your life is from 50s on. Vata energy starts to increase. It makes us lighter, drier, and a little more spacey.

A Realistic Way to Begin

To sum it up, the world is constantly giving you signals about what to do to find balance. You've been introduced to the ideas of Kapha, Pitta, and Vata and how these energies play out in the seasons and times of day—our external world. From here, you'll begin to learn about the sources of your own imbalances and feel confident about stepping into the next phase of your self-care—with well-informed, specific lifestyle shifts.

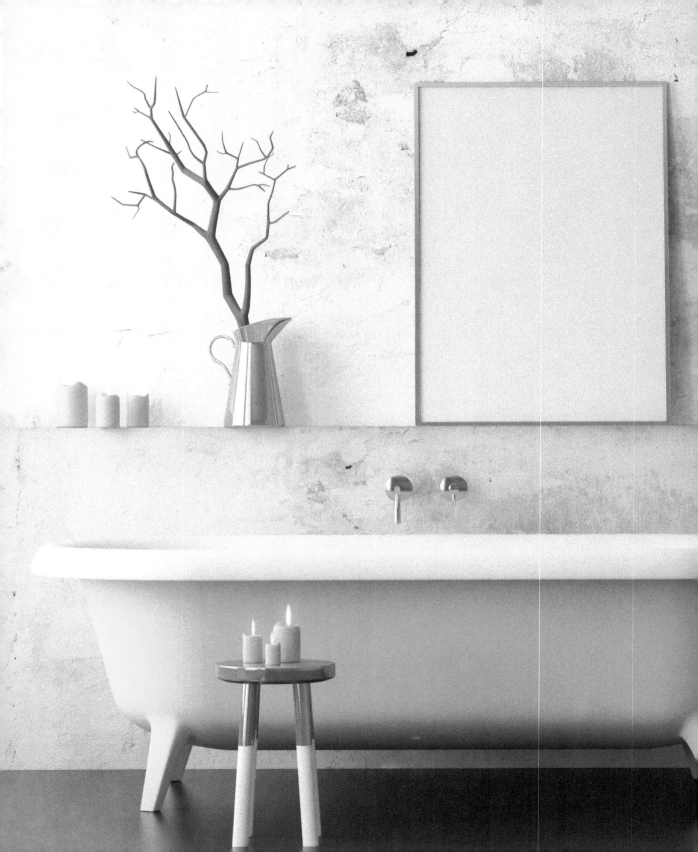

2

AYURVEDA
AND YOU

Now that you have a basic understanding of Ayurveda in the world, it's time to bring it home to yourself. The same seasonal and time-of-day concepts can be used to illustrate how we may get off track. Too much Kapha, too much Pitta, or too much Vata in us will upset the delicate balance at work. So, the question is *why*? Why would we have "too much" of any one dosha?

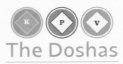

The Doshas

Kapha, Pitta, and Vata. Ayurveda calls these three different energies *doshas*. Dosha, roughly translated, means "fault." And when a dosha is very obvious, it can be because it is out of balance. Going forward, you'll look at how the doshas play out in you, as your Ayurvedic constitution.

Take this quiz to find out which dosha or doshas influence you the most.

FINDING YOUR DOSHA QUIZ

My body type is:
- **A.** Slender
- **B.** Athletic
- **C.** Voluptuous

My hair is:
- **A.** Thin, frizzy
- **B.** Curly, rough, or poker straight
- **C.** Thick, shiny

My eyes are:
- **A.** Almond shaped, dark
- **B.** Piercing, blue, hazel, or gray
- **C.** Round and dark or clear green

My mouth:
- **A.** Is thin, with colorless lips
- **B.** Has a sharp upper lip
- **C.** Is round with full lips

My nose is:
- **A.** Long or boney
- **B.** Triangular
- **C.** Round, with full nostrils

My skin:
- **A.** Tends to dry or ashy
- **B.** Tends to sensitive or irritated
- **C.** Tends to oily or clammy

My weight is:
- **A.** Easy to lose, hard to gain
- **B.** Easy to lose, easy to gain or steady
- **C.** Easy to gain, hard to lose

My stamina is:
- **A.** Weak
- **B.** Middle of the road
- **C.** Strong

My muscles are:
- **A.** Thin and ropey
- **B.** Defined and well-proportioned
- **C.** Thick and strong

My appetite is:
- **A.** Irregular
- **B.** Strong
- **C.** Medium

My cravings lean toward:
A. Crunchy and salty
B. Sour and spicy
C. Sweet and creamy

My sleep is:
A. Short, I wake easily
B. Medium-length, I sleep well
C. Long, I wake up sluggish

I walk:
A. Fast
B. With forceful steps
C. Slow

My memory is such that I:
A. Learn quickly, forget quickly
B. Learn quickly, forget slowly
C. Learn slowly, forget slowly

My job status is:
A. Self-employed; I like independence
B. The boss; I like to be in charge
C. Employed; I'm happy to be a "team player"

At a party, I am:
A. A social butterfly, or I don't show up
B. The life of the party
C. A great host/hostess

I like to be:
A. Interested
B. Respected
C. Trusted

My natural inclinations are:
A. Artistic, musical
B. Business-like, ambitious
C. Friendly, honest

My style icon is:
A. Emma Stone
B. Rihanna
C. Sofia Vergara

COUNT UP YOUR *A*'S, *B*'S, AND *C*'S

Mostly *A*'s = **Vata**

Mostly *B*'s = **Pitta**

Mostly *C*'s = **Kapha**

Mostly *A*'s, some *B*'s = **Vata-Pitta**

Mostly *B*'s some *A*'s = **Pitta-Vata**

Mostly *B*'s, some *C*'s = **Pitta-Kapha**

Mostly *C*'s, some *B*'s = **Kapha-Pitta**

Mostly *A*'s, some *C*'s = **Vata-Kapha**

Mostly *C*'s, some *A*'s = **Kapha-Vata**

Even throughout = **tridoshic**
(if this is you, follow the guidelines for whichever season it is)

Healing Imbalance

Here's where we can start to make some connections. Your four-year-old gets yet another cold and misses school? You are diagnosed with acid indigestion in your mid-30s? An elderly family member is starting to become way more forgetful? Keep reading. Now that you understand what is happening, you can take some actions to make these situations occur less frequently or even disappear altogether.

Let's go even deeper. How do we identify if we have a lot of Pitta? Our next section will shine a light on this. Each dosha has certain physical and mental/emotional traits. Unfortunately, many people, if they have heard about their doshas at all, have only heard about the negative aspects. There's so much more to the story! Each dosha has positive attributes and not-so-positive attributes. Remember the "like increases like" concept? When the characteristics of who you are match up with the characteristics of the world you find yourself in, that's the time when you want to be extra careful about your self-care routines so you can find harmony. This is also where the compassion piece comes in. When you understand yourself (and the people around you) more thoroughly, you can have compassion for the times when you're out of balance and see it for what it is.

NATURE VS. NURTURE

Before we get into a more in-depth look at the doshas, I want to introduce two more Sanskrit words: *prakruti* and *vikruti*.

Prakruti is what we were born as—the combination of doshas that developed when we were in our mamas' bellies. That will not change. And in our most healthy state, we are that same combination, in balance. Think of this as the "nature" aspect of who we are. **Vikruti** is different. Vikruti is our current state, which could be in or out of balance.

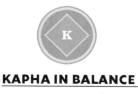

KAPHA IN BALANCE
Physical

Kapha, you're up first. For starters, think about the elements at play here: earth and water. The shape of earth is round. In my initial assessment of my clients, I am just looking at their face and body type. I know they have some Kapha dosha when I see the round shape, like Earth itself. Round eyes, a roundness to the face, a roundness to the lips and the hairline. And there is a connected-to-the-earth quality to their bodies—their frames are a little bigger and sturdier, their walk is a little slower. The women are often curvier; that's the round shape. Water is at play here, too, though, so think about flowing, like hair. Kapha hair is thick, usually dark (that's the earth), and shiny. That goes for the hair on top of the head and often eyebrows and eyelashes. Eyes are usually dark (earth) or clear green (water). Their bones are strong, so that means that their teeth are white, the tips of their nails are usually thick and white. They have great stamina, and they are very fertile. Kapha girls might develop breasts earlier than their classmates, and their menstrual cycle is usually regular and longer, with heavy, red blood. Kapha boys are bigger, and stronger than their classmates. Need some visuals? For women, think Beyoncé, Sofía Vergara, Oprah Winfrey. Men: Shaquille O'Neal, Dwayne Johnson, Jason Momoa. You get the picture, yes?

KAPHA IN BALANCE
Mental and Emotional

What comes to mind for you when someone is described as "earthy"? When I ask this question in my trainings, answers such as "grounded" come back. Yup. "Loyal." Yup. "Trustworthy, honest, friendly." Yup, yup, and yup. To that list, I will add kind, sensitive, and nurturing. Kapha people are great listeners and won't tell your secrets. They learn slowly, but don't forget. Your Kapha friend will remember to call you (not text) on your birthday or your anniversary. They are the friend you want to hang with when you've had a rough day because their presence is so comforting. They won't ask too many questions; they'll just be there. They will make you your favorite dinner, and they will make sure there is dessert. They will give you a big, warm hug, not air-kiss, and you will want to hang on—which is fine with them! They are sensual, tactile people, and comfortable with physical affection. Their easygoing nature makes everyone around them feel calmer. They naturally gravitate toward children, animals, and plants. Their home is comfy, and their refrigerator and cabinets (and bookshelves and drawers) are usually full. Professionally, they make great pediatricians, veterinarians, stay-at-home moms or dads, massage therapists, and social workers.

So, if your mom is a pediatrician and has a lovely curvy figure and shiny hair, or if your dad played football in college and gives great hugs, chances are good you have some Kapha in you.

KAPHA OUT OF BALANCE
Physical

Kapha people like to eat, enjoy life, and sleep soundly. If their Kapha gets too high, they might find that they have gained weight, their skin or hair gets greasy, or their physical appearance is messy. The other dis-eases usually involve being congested or stuck in some way. Wet colds and coughs, lymphoma or fibroids, edema. (All women, when they are pregnant, get more Kapha.) Other issues can be asthma, sluggish digestion, and hypothyroidism. There are more, of course, but that gives you an idea of what to look out for.

KAPHA OUT OF BALANCE
Mental and Emotional

Kapha people who are out of balance can suffer from depression and codependence, and they can become overly sensitive or stubborn. Kapha people love to help out but can be smothering when out of balance. If you're the type of person who stays in a job when you're miserable (because you love your coworker) or stays in your apartment when it makes you miserable (because you're close to the dog park and you have three dogs) or stays with your partner when you are ready to move on (because you don't want to hurt their feelings), then keep reading.

Kapha Imbalances: What to Do?

Kapha, physically, you need to shake yourselves up and get sweaty. Try the new boxing-Pilates-trampoline hybrid class, or just lace up your sneakers, put on some dance music in your headphones, get out in the fresh air, and run around until you're out of breath! For my yogis, add a few extra handstands and twisting poses, and do a little more Breath of Fire and a little less Savasana.

Mentally and emotionally, you need to shake yourself up and get unattached. Take a different route to work, or take a weekend away someplace you've never been. You're always doing for others, so go book a deep-tissue or lymphatic drainage massage and get some circulation going. Acupuncture also gets things unstuck. There is a more in-depth plan on page 115.

Kapha Self-Affirmation

I have the power to change, starting now.

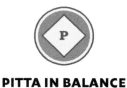

PITTA IN BALANCE
Physical

Pitta people, you're up next. First thing to remember is that Pitta has heat. If you already have heat, and like increases like, then less sun is going to be better for you. Skin that doesn't do as well in the sun is usually relatively light in complexion, or has reddish or yellowish undertones. Doesn't matter the race—if the red or yellow undertones are there, that's Pitta skin. And with light skin, there are usually light eyes. Pitta eyes can be those laser-beam blue eyes, or hazel or green. Their hair is wiry or poker straight, and again, has reddish or yellowish undertones. Their frames are medium, and they often have an athletic build. The shape I look for in my evaluation is a triangle. It might be in the widow's peak of their hairline, the triangle of their nose, a heart-shaped face, a sharpness to their upper lip or eyebrows, or broad shoulders with a tapered waist. For women, think Michelle Obama, Madonna, Michelle Rodriguez. For men, think Liam Hemsworth, Cristiano Ronaldo, Kanye West.

PITTA IN BALANCE
Mental and Emotional

Pitta people are smart. Their *agni*, or digestive fire, is strong in both their bellies and their minds. They like to "get it" and will have the discipline to stay with something until they do. They have that light and brightness, so there is a natural charisma to them, and they can be very charming and persuasive. Your Pitta friend is the one who tells you that you're coming out dancing on a Monday night, you say no because you have an early meeting the next morning . . . but they "won't take no for an answer," and next thing you know it's 3:00 a.m. and you're wondering how you got there.

Pitta personalities are great leaders and speakers, and they are comfortable in the spotlight. Professionally, they can be great movie stars, rock stars, politicians, lawyers, salespeople, pilots, and surgeons—jobs in which you need to walk in and take over with confidence. Pitta people like earthly things. They want uber cool apartments and the latest tech toys.

So, if your mom is a surgeon who does triathlons or your dad is a CEO and the life of the party, you might have inherited some Pitta dosha.

PITTA OUT OF BALANCE
Physical

Out of balance Pitta is usually due to an excess of heat. In the body, this can create an acidic system, so Pitta people can suffer from acid indigestion, acid reflux, and heartburn. Pitta people can also be prone to autoimmune issues like eczema (usually red and moist), rheumatoid arthritis, colitis, and IBS. Their skin is super sensitive, so rosacea, hives, acne, and even excess sweating and body odor are common for someone with out-of-balance Pitta. Hot air rises, and all that heat in the head may make them go gray or bald quite young. They drive themselves hard in all that they do, so they may have injuries of overuse in their bodies. Liver issues like cirrhosis or jaundice and kidney issues like kidney stones can occur.

PITTA OUT OF BALANCE
Mental and Emotional

Again, too much heat. If you're someone who gets hangry (hungry + angry) on a regular basis, you've got some Pitta in there. With too much fire, Pitta people can get mean, angry, and judgmental. They can be perfectionists and turn into workaholics. Their inherent ambition can turn cutthroat, and their inherent daring can turn them into sensation junkies. (Think bungee jumping, heliskiing, driving too fast, etc.)

Pitta Imbalances: What to Do?

The short answer for physical imbalance is cool it down.

Yes, you need a healthy outlet for that competitive drive, so some kind of intense exercise once or twice a week can be good. Please, for the sake of all of us, balance that out with walks or easy bike rides by the water or in a cool, tree-filled spot. Make sure you don't overheat, and remember that includes both under the sun and in front of computers. Stick with soft, natural fabrics and cooling colors like blue, green, white, and gray.

Mentally, make sure you get days off from work (real days off, not just out-of-office days), do some volunteer work to get out of the me-me-me attitude, and make a lunch date with a friend or two. A little secret about Pitta people: If you can just get into their hearts, they are marshmallows. You should see my Pitta dad with my puppy. He cuddles him constantly and cooks him sweet potatoes.

Pitta Self-Affirmation
I am open to loving and being loved.

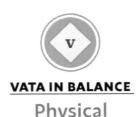

Physical

We will finish with Vata dosha. Physically in balance, my Vata friends are like willow trees in the wind—slender and graceful. They have a cold quality, so some sun is good for them. Their skin is relatively dark, with gray or green undertones. Their hair and eyes are dark, and the shape to look for is oblong—a longer face, almond eyes, and narrow hips and shoulders. Their skin seems poreless, and they are more interested in looking unique than looking trendy. They might be the woman in your yoga class with blue hair and lots of tattoos, or your friend's boyfriend who wears only black and paints his nails silver. Women with a lot of Vata are Billie Eilish, Zendaya, and Selena Gomez. Vata men are Marilyn Manson, Christian Bale, and Chris Rock.

VATA IN BALANCE
Mental and Emotional

When mentally and emotionally in balance, Vata people are otherworldly. By that I mean they are often highly creative and imaginative. They think outside the box with a curious nature and an intensity that often makes them experts in their field. They are artistic, musical, and unusual. They might thrive on alone time, or they might flit about like social butterflies, not lingering too long with anyone. They are spontaneous and adventurous, but they feel best when they balance that with routine and ritual. Spirituality comes naturally to them, and they often are interested in "alternative" lifestyles. Professionally, they can make great writers, artists, scientists, fashion designers, and clergypeople.

So, if your mom is a physics professor who speaks three languages and your father plays the cello and collects books about mythology, you might have inherited some Vata.

VATA OUT OF BALANCE
Physically

When physically out of balance, Vata people can be clumsy and awkward, like they don't fully inhabit their bodies. They can get frail, anemic, or dizzy if they don't have proper nutrition. Their skin and hair become dry and ashy-looking. That same dryness causes constipation and gas. Vata is associated with the nervous system, so Parkinson's disease, tics, and tremors can appear. They are chilled easily, and they might develop hypothyroid or hyperthyroid conditions or amenorrhea if high Vata is left untreated. Infertility or low bone density can be an issue. Their joints may crack, and they might be prone to breaking bones.

VATA OUT OF BALANCE
Mental and Emotional

Mentally, there is such a thing as too much space! Vata minds are super quick and highly intelligent; left unchecked, that can turn into anxiety and fear. Out of balance, they are forgetful, unreliable, or obsessive. Autism and spectrum disorders fall under Vata, as do ADD and ADHD. Going further, high Vata can be the cause of bipolar disorder, paranoia, and OCD.

Vata Imbalances: What to Do?

My advice for my clients with high Vata is to treat yourself like you would treat a baby. You would not want to let a baby get cold or overheated. You wouldn't play music too loudly or turn lights up too brightly in a baby's room. You would swaddle the baby in soft, natural colors and fabrics and give them something interesting to play with. Their food would be nourishing and warm, and you would make sure their bath wasn't too hot and their skin was well moisturized. Voila! A Vata-balancing protocol!

Vata Self-Affirmation
I am so taken care of.

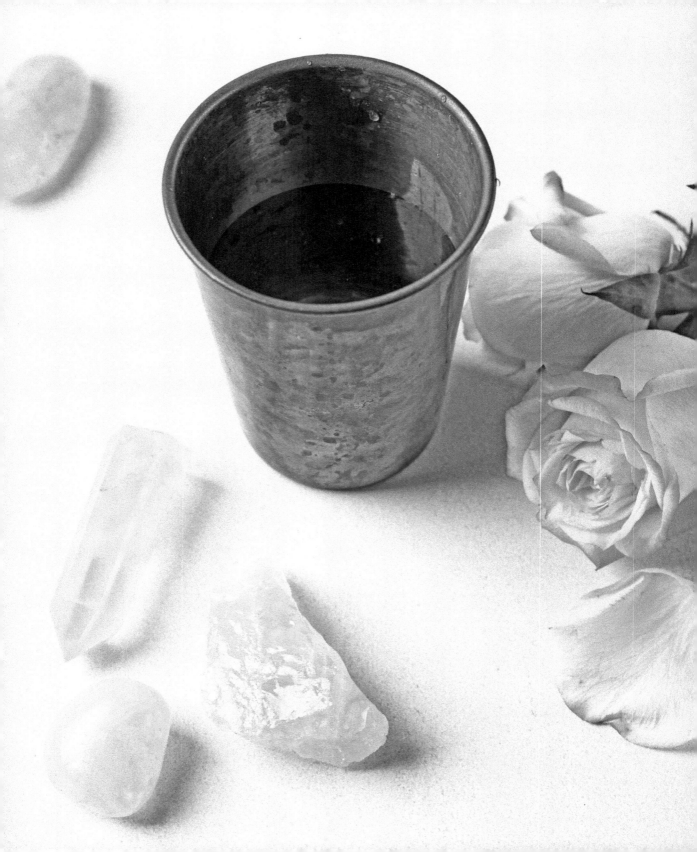

3

MODERN AYURVEDA LIFESTYLE: RITUALS, PRINCIPLES, AND PRACTICES

Now you should have a better idea of your constitution, both physical and mental. Great! Let's move on to some more practical information about how to stay in balance, or how to start making some adjustments if you've identified imbalances. This chapter will cover Ayurvedic theory regarding what to eat, how to eat it, and when to eat it. We will also cover some simple remedies and tools for daily and seasonal wellness made from things you might already have in your kitchen or bathroom cabinet. Anything mentioned that you don't have should be easily available on the Internet.

I've kept an eye toward budget and practicality with all recommendations. If new stuff isn't in the budget right now, no worries! Do what you can, and maybe you'll get to it in the future. As I said before, even the small changes add up.

A FEW WORDS ABOUT FOOD "RULES"

Many of my clients and students have a past history or current struggle with eating disorders. If this is you, dear reader, please know that what we discuss in this chapter is Ayurvedic theory around what, where, how much, and when to eat. I do my best to give you a complete picture as we go, so you have the opportunity to see that there are always exceptions to every "rule." That being said, there can be certain triggers around food talk for some people. I firmly believe the best way to eat is in a way that makes you feel good and satisfied, and keeps your body and mind working well. If what you're currently eating does that continue! If you're consuming food in a way that makes you feel unhealthy and unhappy, I encourage you to seek out professional help. You don't have to try to shift that on your own. See page 158 for a list of resources.

Gratitude as the Main Ingredient

I live in New York City, and eating out can be very (very!) expensive. Once a week, I treat myself to lunch at an organic restaurant near my yoga center. I get a salad, and it costs around 12 bucks. I enjoy it, it's delicious, and it makes me feel good.

Let's acknowledge that having a choice to "eat better" is a choice of privilege. So, when I talk about choosing organic quinoa and baby kale over macaroni and cheese (not that there isn't a time and place for mac and cheese!), I do so with the knowledge that if we can afford to make changes, we have a certain level of economic security. Basic needs are taken care of, which is not the case for everyone. *All the more reason to have gratitude for what's in our bowl.* I invite you to put the book down for a moment and just be grateful for the blessings in your life. Take a gratitude pause, and let it sink in.

Some of us have been raised with cultural associations around certain foods. One of my best friends is Italian, and we travel together. If we get delayed or something goes awry in our travels, she says, "I need a bowl of pasta." For her, it's comfort food and makes her feel more grounded and calm. In that case, it doesn't matter if it's the food recommended for her dosha in that moment. It makes her feel good, so it is perfect!

That actually is part of Ayurvedic theory. You never want to become so strict about food that it becomes stressful. For that matter, any of the Ayurvedic recommendations are just that—recommendations. You shouldn't become so rigid about any of it that it causes more stress. If you go to your best friend's house for dinner and they make you a dinner that doesn't align with the way you usually eat, bless it, eat some, and thank your friend for their efforts. The next day you can eat whatever you choose. If you're in a country other than your own and they're eating differently than you're used to, try some! The local food is often the most seasonal and expertly prepared. Okay. All good? Let's get into it.

Eating Principles

"When food is wrong, medicine is of no use. When food is right, medicine is of no need."

— *Charaka Samhita*, primary ancient Ayurvedic text

What's great about food these days is that, in many places, everything is available all the time. What's not so great about food these days is that, in many places, everything is available all the time. You live in Maine and you want a pineapple in December? You can find it! You live in Texas and you want apples in May? You can get those. You can end up eating out of season, not to mention that we are adding pollution to the atmosphere and using up natural resources flying pineapples in from Hawaii and apples from Washington state. When I was doing my first Ayurvedic training, my teacher brought the whole class to the farmers' market and said, "See what they have? Eat that!" But how do we know what to do when we don't have access to a farmers' market or we don't have time to get to one?

Ayurveda gives you great guidelines.

Six Tastes

The whole food system in Ayurveda is based on the *shadrasa*, or six tastes. The six tastes are sweet, salty, sour, pungent, bitter, and astringent. And, going back to our five elements—earth, water, fire, wind, and space—each of the six tastes is associated with two elements. Each has a certain effect on you—whether it is cooling or heating, makes you feel heavier or lighter, or makes you feel drier or more lubricated. Everyone needs all six tastes, just in varying percentages. Each dosha has three tastes that are most beneficial, and if you identify with that dosha, those tastes should make up a greater percentage of your diet while the remaining three tastes should make up a lesser percentage.

- **If you have a lot of Kapha,** follow the Kapha guidelines most of the time, adding some Vata guidelines in autumn and early winter and some Pitta guidelines in summer.
- **If you have a lot of Pitta,** follow the Pitta guidelines most of the time, adding some Vata guidelines in autumn and early winter and some Kapha guidelines in late winter and spring.
- **If you have a lot of Vata,** follow the Vata guidelines most of the time, adding some Pitta guidelines in summer and some Kapha guidelines in late winter and spring.

Let's look at these tastes more closely.

▪ SWEET

When we think of sweetness, what comes to mind? Sugar, sure, but let's consider unprocessed sweet foods. Some of my favorites fall into this category: coconut, sweet potatoes, and blueberries. Most nuts, fruits, and root veggies go here. What else? Ayurveda also puts whole grains in this category, as well as some dairy products. Blue cheese and other strong cheeses don't go here, and neither does yogurt. (I will explain that when we discuss the sour taste.) However, ghee, milk, cream, cottage cheese, ricotta, and other soft cheeses do.

The sweet taste is associated with the elements of earth and water. It is cooling, lubricating, and heavy in quality. Its lubricating and heavy qualities are good for Vata dosha. Its cooling and heavy qualities are good for Pitta. It's not so good for Kapha, because Kapha is already heavy, cold, and lubed up and is associated with earth and water as well. Remember: Like increases like, and opposites balance. So Kapha people, this doesn't mean you shouldn't have the sweet taste in your diet; it just means it should be minimized. Vata and Pitta people, I will give you advice that I often give my Vata and Pitta clients when they're out of balance in any way—eat a sweet potato and get back to me.

GOOD FOR: Vata, Pitta   **MINIMIZE FOR:** Kapha

▪ SALTY
....

I'm a big fan. There is a shorter list here. Sea salt, rock salt, and some veggies have naturally occurring saline in them. Celery, seaweed, and artichokes all have around 75 milligrams of sodium per serving. The salty taste is associated with water and fire. Think about sea salt; it comes from water but needs heat to be solidified. It's heating, heavy, and lubricating. Don't you find when you feel heavier when you overdo salt? That's because salt makes us retain water. Since it's heating and lubricating, it's not so good for Pitta. Since it's heavy and lubricating, it's not so good for Kapha. But my Vata people, salt is better for you because it is water and fire—it's helpful to balance out all that wind and space! That doesn't give you permission to finish your giant bag of cheese popcorn (more on popcorn later); it just means that adding a sprinkle of Himalayan salt or sea salt to your sweet potato is a good idea.

GOOD FOR: Vata   **MINIMIZE FOR:** Pitta, Kapha

▪ SOUR
....

Generally, people think of citrus fruits first when they think of sour foods. And that's correct. Citrus fruit belongs in this category, as do all fermented foods, including miso, kombucha, tempeh, soy sauce, alcohol, vinegar, yogurt, kimchi, and pickles. The sour taste is associated with earth and fire. Everything on the list comes from the earth, sure, but has a flavorful kick to it. The sour taste is heating, lubricating, and light. Despite its lightness, it's best for Vata because of the heating and moistening properties. It's too heating for Pitta, and too lubricating for Kapha. Again, this doesn't mean Pitta or Kapha people shouldn't have it at all; it just means they should indulge less frequently.

GOOD FOR: Vata   **MINIMIZE FOR:** Pitta, Kapha

EATING FOR BALANCE

Here's where Ayurveda differs from other food trends. I have Pitta clients who come to me in the summer and say, "I don't know why I am having diarrhea! I am being so healthy—I'm drinking all this ginger kombucha!" You're having diarrhea because you're drinking all that ginger kombucha. Ginger is heating, kombucha is heating, and it's making your tummy boil over.

▪ PUNGENT

Pungent includes all of your hot, spicy foods. Right away, you know it ain't gonna be the right thing for Pitta—but Pitta people, you *love* your hot spicy foods, don't you? I get it—I was a "hot sauce in my bag" woman for many years. I would actually take the pepper mill out of the server's hands (how Pitta!) because I just wanted to cover my food with pepper and I felt bad for them standing there, grinding away, with me saying, "More, more, please!" This category includes garlic, radishes, ground ginger (fresh ginger is sweet and pungent; ground ginger is more purely pungent), tomatoes, and hot peppers. We know fire is one of the elements, and air makes fire bigger, so the pungent taste is related to fire and air. It's heating, drying, and light—best for Kapha, not good for Pitta and Vata.

GOOD FOR: Kapha   **MINIMIZE FOR:** Pitta, Vata

BALANCE AND CRAVINGS

I used to *love* spicy food! The hotter the better! But it wasn't good for me—I have a lot of dryness, and it made me drier, and when I don't eat properly, my childhood eczema comes back. I vowed to slow down on the spice considerably about five years ago. And guess what. I lost the taste for it. I no longer want it. I still like flavorful food—cumin, coriander, turmeric, and fennel get a lot of play when I cook—but the fiery stuff is no longer interesting to me. Confession: I'm still a popcorn addict, though, which is also not great for me; it's dry, and I already have dryness (Vata), and it's acidic, and I have a lot of acidity (Pitta). One time I asked my teacher, Dr. Lad, why we are drawn to things that put us out of balance. His answer was that when the system is full of *ama*, or toxins, you don't make good decisions. Ama can build up from poor diet or sleep habits, too much work or travel, or even too much stress on the nervous system from loud noises or angry conversations. And think about it: How many times have you been exhausted, had an argument with your partner or family, or stayed out way past your bedtime and ended up reaching for food you wouldn't normally be drawn to or having more alcohol, pizza, or ice cream than you planned? I usually reach for a bag of popcorn when I have stayed up too late or have not eaten properly during the day and have nighttime munchies. Along the same lines, when you are taking care of yourself, getting proper food and sleep, not working too much, and spending time with people you care for who support and love you, you will find that another drink, bag of candy, hot sauce, or a giant bag of popcorn is less attractive.

• BITTER

The bitter taste is found in leafy greens and bitter lettuces: baby kale and arugula, dandelion greens (so cleansing!), romaine and Boston lettuce, and radicchio. Aloe vera also goes in this category, as do barley and burdock root. Spinach and chard do not, though. They are both acidic, so they fit better in the pungent category, which means that, unlike true bitter greens, they are not good for Pitta. The bitter taste is made up of wind and space. It's cooling, drying, and light.

GOOD FOR: Pitta, Kapha   **MINIMIZE FOR:** Vata

LIKE INCREASES LIKE

Many of my Vata clients initially come to me complaining of always being cold or stiff and dry in November or December and then say they can't understand why, because they are being so healthy and starting every day off with a big green juice! This is fine for them in 85°F weather, but not a good choice for a frigid winter day.

• ASTRINGENT

Astringency. What exactly is it? We find it in dried legumes, lentils, apples, quinoa, tofu, and pomegranate. The best way to describe the taste is this way—some of us, when we were kids, couldn't swallow pills. That was me, and when I needed aspirin, my parents used to crush it up and put it in pudding or applesauce. Inevitably, though, one piece wouldn't get crushed enough, and I would end up biting down on it. Oof. I can still taste it today. If you weren't one of those kids, but you cook, think of the time you made lentils but you didn't quite cook them long enough, and then you tried to eat them. You bit down on that grainy, icky taste. Same thing; it makes your lips curl inward and your eyes squint. While we are on it, all medicine is considered astringent. It's made up of the elements of earth and wind. It is cooling, drying, and heavy. Astringent tastes are best for Pitta, and Kapha as well. They're very cleansing.

GOOD FOR: Pitta, Kapha   **MINIMIZE FOR:** Vata

Okay; let's sum up what is best for each dosha.

- **Kapha:** pungent, bitter, and astringent
- **Pitta:** sweet, bitter, and astringent
- **Vata:** sweet, sour, and salty

Top Food Recommendations

Here are the top 10 Ayurvedic food recommendations for optimal eating conditions.

1. **Ayurveda doesn't recommend too much raw food for anyone.** It can be difficult to digest, especially for delicate Vata digestion. Everyone has a set level of agni, or digestive fire, which can be improved or challenged by eating habits. Much of Ayurveda is based on how good your digestion is—both physically and mentally. You could be eating the healthiest diet in the world, but if you are not digesting well, it doesn't matter. Likewise, you could be listening to the wisest lecture in the world and not understanding or retaining (digesting) any of it! Raw food is cold, so it requires a lot of agni to get the digestive process going. Cooked food is easier for your system, as the cell walls have been broken down a little before you ingest it. A big salad for lunch in warm weather is a great choice. The sun is very strong, so your digestive fire is improved. In cold weather, try to stick to warm or hot food. That doesn't mean the food should be limp and overcooked; it should be just properly cooked with good spices that help the digestive process.

2. **Because your agni is strongest in Pitta time, Ayurvedic theory says lunch should be your biggest meal.** And many countries do come to a full stop at lunch. But what if you have 15 minutes and need to eat at your desk? That's fine, but put your computer to sleep. Get off the phone. Give yourself those 15 minutes without distraction to eat mindfully. If you have longer, the same principle applies, and if you can take a gentle walk after lunch for a few minutes to get some fresh air, even better!

3. **Chew well.** According to both Ayurveda and Western science, digestion begins in the mouth. Give your agni some help!

4. **Don't drink too much water or other beverages while you eat.** Too much liquid dampens your digestive fire. Try to hydrate well at least an hour before you eat, and wait at least an hour after to drink again. If you feel like you need to drink a lot while you're eating, chances are you're either very dehydrated or your food is too salty or spicy for you. Your body is trying to cool you down! Iced drinks are not recommended, as ice—you guessed it—cools down agni too much.

5. **Combine your food properly.** Western nutrition is mindful of this as well. Ayurveda advises not to eat fruit in combination with other foods, as fruit digests more quickly than other foods. If another food is blocking the fruit from making it out of your belly, fermentation can occur, leading to gas and bloating. This means the mango lassi (a mango and yogurt smoothie) at your local Indian restaurant is not Ayurvedic. An Ayurvedic lassi is made with slightly watered-down, runny yogurt and some digestive spices. If you're not vegetarian, don't combine two kinds of protein (e.g., chicken and fish, or bacon and eggs) in one meal. Ayurveda advises simple, flavorful, fresh, in-season meals.

6. **Freshness is key.** Ayurvedic theory is not a fan of leftovers. Leftovers are considered *tamasic*, which means "lifeless or stale." Likewise, canned food and frozen food is not considered optimal.

7. **Animal protein is a hotly debated topic.** Here's what Ayurvedic theory said 4,000 or so years ago: For Vata, if you're eating meat, choose dark meat, oily fish, whole eggs, and full-fat dairy. For Pitta and Kapha, stick to white meat, white fish, egg whites, and low-fat dairy. Ayurveda was big on milk and milk products as a source of vegetarian protein. As you know, the modern milk industry is very different from what it was in ancient times, and there are wonderful plant-based milks out there. Again, I never insist food rules are carved in stone. Use your judgment, and stay informed so you can make responsible choices. If you've been eating a lot of animal protein, try cutting down a bit. Vegetarian cooking is so innovative! See chapter 4 for some ideas.

8. **If you are not cooking for any reason and you're buying your food from a restaurant or prepared food in a supermarket, make eye contact with the person giving you your meal.** This person, in the moment, is handing you your energy and sustenance. Be gracious and say hello, please, and thank you, and if you're in a restaurant, tip well if the service was good or you stayed a long time.

9. **Try not to eat too much or too often.** It takes some time for the brain to register fullness, and in the meantime, we can have seconds or thirds. Slow down. As mentioned, chew well. Don't speak too much while you're eating. Try to eat in a restful environment, if possible, so your system is in rest-and-digest mode. When your nervous system is on high alert, blood moves from your organs to your limbs (arms and legs), so you can fight or flee. This results in less energy for digestion.

10. **Don't forget to pray or offer gratitude in your own way for your meal.** One of the ancient texts says that our bodies are "food, rearranged." Let's remember to be grateful for what we have access to, whether it is a "perfect" meal or not.

CONSIDERATION

I can't tell you how many Pitta people I have counseled who have thrown their Pitta out of whack by starting their mornings with a popular concoction of hot water with lemon, ginger, and apple cider vinegar or cayenne. One client, Ines, was pure Pitta and doing shots of apple cider vinegar for her body aches because she heard it was good for inflammation, and she then wondered why her rheumatoid arthritis was flaring up.

Yikes. Oftentimes, Pitta people have issues with acidity in the stomach and read somewhere that some combo of those substances is "good for digestion." This is true, but not for Pitta digestion. Pitta digestion needs cooling. Vata digestion needs warming, and Kapha digestion needs heating. Pitta folks looking for a morning tonic do better with a glass of water, a splash of soothing aloe juice, and a bit of cooling mint.

Drinking Principles

Ayurvedic theory also applies to what, where, and how much you drink. One of the main principles is to limit drinking too much when you eat, as it can put out your digestive fire. Try to stay well hydrated during the time you are not eating, so it doesn't feel as urgent to drink at mealtimes.

Ayurveda also encourages you to watch your food combos with smoothies. The practice doesn't recommend adding nuts to fruits (e.g., a banana smoothie with almond butter), nor does it recommend milk with fruit (e.g., a blueberry smoothie with yogurt).

Here are a few more recommendations with regard to beverages.

Water

So many of us don't get enough water and get dehydrated, which can lead to fuzzy thinking, muscle cramps, constipation, and other unpleasant imbalances. Increase your water intake, but skip the ice: It isn't recommended for any dosha. Warm beverages are recommended, especially in the morning. Try keeping a mug of warm water near you throughout the day, and take small sips regularly.

Alcohol

Beer, wine, and spirits should be used in moderation—if at all. It's a substance that can substantially alter your physical and mental capabilities, so use it wisely. If an occasional drink is okay for you, here are some guidelines.

- Kapha, you're pretty hardy, but heavy liquor or sweet mixes will make you drag for days. If you are drinking, stay away from the sugary blended drinks and dark whiskeys. Stick to clear liquor with some seltzer and lemon.

- Pitta, the dark stuff will increase the acid in your body, and heartburn and inflammation can be intense. In addition, those loosened inhibitions might make you loud, rude, or bossy, so monitor that and limit yourself accordingly. Try to skip the beer and red wine, and stick to a glass of white wine or clear liquor. Add a bit of juice to your drink; pomegranate or coconut is best.

- Vata, your constitution is so delicate. Some red wine with dinner is okay; it helps digestion and might be slightly calming, but limit yourself to a small glass. Red wine dehydrates and decreases the likelihood of sleeping well, which you need for optimal health.

Beverage Trends: What About a Matcha-Kombucha Latte Smoothie?

Here's the Ayurvedic take on:

KOMBUCHA

- Okay for Kapha (especially spicy flavors like ginger)
- Not recommended for Pitta (it's too sour)
- Best for Vata (any flavor)

MATCHA

- Best for Kapha (without milk)
- Okay for Pitta and Vata (occasionally, with milk)

LATTES OF ALL TYPES (CHAI, MOCHA, TURMERIC)

- Not recommended for Kapha
- Okay for Pitta
- Best for Vata (as they're usually more milk than anything else)

COCONUT WATER

- Not recommended for Kapha
- Best for Pitta
- Okay for Vata (in the summer)

GREEN JUICE

- Okay for Kapha (if it's without added sweet fruit)
- Best for Pitta
- Not recommended for Vata

PROTEIN DRINKS

- Not recommended for Kapha
- Okay for Pitta (when the fire is raging and dinner is hours away)

- ◆ Okay for Vata (as a supplement to increase protein intake, especially if vegetarian or vegan)

ENERGY DRINKS

- ◆ Okay for Kapha (if you're really dragging and green tea and/or a treadmill is nowhere close)
- ◆ Not recommended for Pitta or Vata (can promote insomnia)

WHAT ABOUT COFFEE?

Coffee belongs under the "bitter" umbrella. Many of my clients look at me in their initial consult and say (fearfully), "You're not taking away my coffee, are you?" or (menacingly), "You're not taking away my coffee are you?!" If you love your coffee, have it—just observe its effect on you. If it gives you the shakes, loose stool, or an acidic stomach, that's a sign that your system doesn't tolerate it very well. I suggest that if you love it, have it in the morning but not on an empty stomach. Hydrate well with water first, then have your coffee with breakfast. Get the best coffee you can afford or find, preferably organic, as nonorganic coffee is grown with a lot of pesticides. For both Vata and Pitta types, it's best to add either dairy milk or nondairy milk. Kapha folks can do black coffee, but don't overdo it, as it can be tough on the adrenals. Try to swap out your afternoon coffee for tea (herbal if possible, or green if you need a little caffeine), or forego caffeine altogether, as it can disturb your sleep.

Digestion: What If I'm Not Pooping?

I warned you we were going to talk about poop. Here goes. You gotta do it. Every morning. And not because you're chugging a triple espresso or using chemical laxatives. Oftentimes, if you are not moving your bowels in the morning, it is because your colon is dehydrated. If you have been sleeping for six to eight hours, your body needs hydration. I have gotten into the habit of filling a 24-ounce mason jar in the morning with filtered, room-temperature water (heated is good, too), then adding a squeeze of lemon juice or apple cider vinegar in the colder months or aloe juice and fresh mint in warmer months. I make sure I finish it all before I even think about eating; and I don't eat breakfast until *after* I use the bathroom.

If you haven't slept enough, or woke up several times during the night, your digestion won't work as well and you may end up feeling constipated. This is all the more reason to get enough sleep and not rush through your mornings. Rushing is not going to help. Constipation is a terrible feeling and means that ama (toxins) are building up in your system. You should be moving your bowels before you eat anything in the morning. If you're struggling with that, I recommend trying *triphala*. It's an Ayurvedic compound made from three different dried and powdered fruits—Amalaki, Bibhitaki, and Haritaki. It can be helpful for all doshas, and the powder is better than the pills. You should taste it, so your tongue and mind register the taste and start the healing process. Start with ½ teaspoon in warm water before bed. If you get the pills, even if it says take two on the label, just take one. See how your system does with it for a month or so before you shift the dose. It should not interfere with any Western medication you may be on.

Triphala has a slight laxative quality, and it is loaded with vitamin C and antioxidants, so it also supports your immune system. Most important, it's not habit-forming, and it's designed to improve your digestive system so you can start to regulate your bowel movements. And don't worry! It's not going to work so fast or so strongly that you are on your way to work and all of a sudden you have a major emergency on your hands. It helps out in a gentle way.

WHAT IF I'M POOPING A LOT?

Isn't that a good thing? Actually, it's not. If you move your bowels in the morning and then have to go 20 minutes after you eat every meal, it's not so good for you. It often means that your food isn't digesting properly, and nutrients are not being absorbed. If your stool is loose and runny for longer than a day or so, please check in with your doctor. Ayurveda doesn't recommend use of diarrhea blockers: That's another way of treating the symptom, not the cause. Diarrhea is a Pitta condition, so shift your diet to include more cooling foods and see if that helps.

Cooking

When I was doing my very first Ayurvedic training, one of my classmates raised their hand and said, "I like to make a big pot of soup on Sunday night. I eat some and freeze the rest, and then take it out each night for the next few days and reheat it. Should I be buying food out on those nights instead?" My teacher, Sri Maya Tiwari, said, "It's always better to eat eat food that you've prepared than to buy food." My friend said, "I don't have time to cook every night," and Maya replied, "Do the best you can." I love to pass this on. It would be nice if we could all grow our own produce; pick it each day; have time to clean, prep, and cook it; and eat it in peace. That's not reality for most—especially in our modern world. So do the best you can. If that means freezing and reheating homemade soup or buying food out and adding some balancing spices to it, then so be it.

Spices

While we are on the subject, let's talk about spices because they really are nature's gift to our digestion. Go into your kitchen and take a peek at your spice rack. If everything in there is over a year old, throw it out. You don't need a ton of spices. Here are my favorites. Buy a small quantity of the whole seeds when available, dry roast them in a stainless steel or cast iron pan, and either crush them with a mortar and pestle (the old-school way, very satisfying for getting out frustrations) or grind 'em up in a coffee grinder (effective, but not as fun). And for those of you with children, they'll get a kick out of using the mortar and pestle. I use a big stone one called a *molcajete*.

- **Cumin** Provides great support for digestion, metabolism, and circulation. It may reduce gas and bloating and can help relieve menstrual cramps. It's officially tridoshic, but in the case of high Pitta, reduce its use.

- **Coriander** Cooling and slightly bitter, it's great support for digestion and detoxification. It's also an excellent spice for reducing excess Pitta and may be helpful in relieving allergies. Coriander is tridoshic.

- **Turmeric** This golden beauty has been getting a lot of press from Western science as of late. It gives the nervous system strong support, and it's also antibacterial, antifungal, digestive, and anti-inflammatory. Buy the whole, fresh root for smoothies and soups. Otherwise, the powder is fine. It's become very popular, and is an ingredient in Golden Milk (page 91). It is incredibly soothing for out-of-balance Vata dosha. Access its powers even more with the addition of black pepper. Turmeric is tridoshic.

- **Fennel** This cooling and sweet spice is appropriate for all doshas and known for its digestive support. In fact, you often see a little bowl of fennel seeds offered at the end of an Indian meal. Fennel can be helpful for circulation, has diuretic properties, and can relieve nausea. On long car rides, I bring some seeds to chew on, as they are helpful for relieving motion sickness.

- **Cinnamon** Cinnamon is best for Kapha, excellent for Vata, and okay in small quantities for Pitta. As it is heating, it stimulates circulation. If you crave sugar, brew up a cup of cinnamon tea for after dinner or whenever the craving hits. It's been proven to help reduce cholesterol. It can be soothing for sore throats and can help break up congestion. Buy it whole, and give yourself a good workout pounding into powder! It's a must for oatmeal, baked apples, and curry sauces.

- **Cardamom** Excellent for digestion and circulation. Throw some whole pods into the pot while you're making rice or quinoa. Fun fact—it reduces acidity in coffee, so put a few pods or a pinch of the powder in your coffee filter.

- **Cloves** These are heating, as well as sweet and astringent. Cloves have antibacterial and antifungal properties. They support immunity and powerfully aid circulation.

- **Black Pepper** Heating and pungent, black pepper is not great for Pitta, good in small quantities for Vata, and most appropriate for Kapha. It's stimulating and can boost circulation while reducing phlegm and congestion.

- **Ginger** This spice has heating, sweet, and pungent qualities. The fresh root is better for Vata, and the dried powder is better for Kapha, as it is more pungent. It makes a great tea after a meal for Vata and Kapha. Pitta types do better with peppermint tea.

- **Mint** Cooling, sweet, and supportive for digestion. Great for Pitta and Kapha, it's a bit drying for Vata. It's digestive and stimulating, and it can help with circulation and nausea. It also helps clear sinuses and phlegm. I love fresh mint in smoothies in the summer, and I keep peppermint essential oil with me at all times to sniff as an afternoon pick-me-up or to help relieve headache pain.

Rituals and Practices

In Ayurveda, our daily routines are called *dinacharya*. The way you start your day is so important! It sets the mood and the tone for how the day will go. Don't feel like you have to do all of these rituals every day. Pick the one that resonates with you the most to start off with, and try to incorporate another one after your initial choice becomes second nature.

Morning Sense Cleansing Rituals

Here are some simple actions to get you started in your day feeling calm, grounded, and prepared. Morning practices are more about cleansing and detoxing—starting the day off fresh before the input of food, drink, conversation, and work.

Ayurvedic theory tells us that we stay present with more ease when our senses are working to their full capacity. This ritual helps alert the senses that it's time to wake up.

- ◆ **Sight and touch.** For your sense of sight and touch, cup some cool water in your hands and splash your face a few times.
- ◆ **Taste.** For your sense of taste, brush your teeth with a natural toothbrush and toothpaste, and scrape your tongue with a tongue scraper—they are easy to find online! Use a stainless steel scraper for Pitta and a copper scraper for Vata and Kapha. Clear the ama from the tongue.
- ◆ **Smell.** For your sense of smell, use a neti pot filled with room temperature or warm, filtered water and a tiny pinch of salt to rinse the nostrils. Afterward, take your pinky finger and dip it in sesame oil (for Vata and Kapha) or coconut oil (for Pitta), and rub a tiny bit of oil inside your nostrils.
- ◆ **Hearing.** For your sense of hearing, rinse your hands, dip your finger again in oil, and swirl a little oil gently in your ears, almost like you're giving your ears a massage.

Here's a fun finish. Add ¼ teaspoon triphala to a cup of warm water. Take a mouthful and swirl it around well, then spit it out as hard as you can. Take another mouthful and gargle well, and again spit it out as hard as you can! (If you have access to a yard, this can be done there.) Drink whatever is left. This is designed to get your *udana* moving. Udana is the force that propels us to speak, and it's located in the throat. The idea behind the spitting is to make our truth come out more easily. It can get a little messy in a small sink, but if you have to have a difficult conversation or give a speech in front of a group and you're feeling a little nervous, give it a try!

In Sanskrit, the word for oil is *sneha*.
The same word is used for "love."
Isn't that sweet? Love should feel like
a warm, protective coating.

Morning Tonics

Again, when you wake up, you are usually dehydrated, so you want to hydrate and kindle your agni before eating. Here are some easy formulas for a tonic for each season. If your Kapha is high, stick with the Kapha tonic, regardless of the season, likewise with Pitta and Vata. Each of these will help start your agni up for the day, getting your body prepared to receive nourishment.

▪ KAPHA TONIC

- Heat 16 ounces of water until it just simmers.
- Add a pinch each of dried ginger and black pepper and a big squeeze of lemon. Add a teaspoon of honey at the last minute. Sip slowly while it's still warm.

▪ PITTA TONIC

- Simmer 16 ounces of water for five minutes with one hibiscus tea bag and one dandelion tea bag.
- Let it cool to room temperature, and remove the tea bags.
- Pour your tonic into a mug, and add ½ teaspoon of raw sugar or coconut sugar. Sip slowly as you move into your day.

▪ VATA TONIC

- Simmer 16 ounces of water with ½ teaspoon each of cumin, coriander, and fennel seeds.
- Strain and drink, a few sips at a time, while warm before breakfast. You can finish the rest with your breakfast.
- This tonic is also helpful for female hormone balancing, so if your menstrual cycle is difficult or irregular, you may sip on this formula all day long.

Morning Yoga Practice

Here's a 10-minute yoga practice for each season. Again, if you feel like your Kapha energy is always high and you are trying to balance that out, stay with the Kapha practice no matter the season. If Pitta energy is too high, stay with the Pitta practice, and if Vata energy is too high, stay with the Vata practice.

ⓚ KAPHA MORNING YOGA

1. Start sitting on your heels or on a block or cushion. **A**

2. Rub your palms together vigorously, then reach your arms up in a V for Victory. **B**

3. Fold your four fingers in to the base of their own knuckles, and extend your thumbs up like you're hitchhiking.

4. Begin Breath of Fire, which is similar to a dog panting, but keep your mouth closed and do the breathing through your nose. If you're new to yoga, do this for 30 seconds; if you're more experienced, do it for one minute; and if you're a regular yoga practitioner, you can do this for three minutes. Note: Do not perform Breath of Fire if you're pregnant, have just eaten, or are on the first or second day of your menstrual cycle.

5. At the end, lift your hands up and touch your thumbs above your head with a breath in. Retain your breath in, and take the tip of your tongue up to the soft palate at the roof of your mouth and swallow.

6. Lie down, and let your breath out. Sit for a couple of breaths, then stand up.

7. Do three to five rounds of Sun Salutations (see page 45). **C**

8. Finish up by lying on your back, pulling your knees into your chest **D**, and letting them drop to the left. Take two deep breaths. Let your knees drop to the right, and take two deep breaths. Then squeeze your knees into your chest, rock and roll forward and back a couple times, and come up to sit. Finish by taking your hands to your heart in prayer and chanting "rammmmm" one time. It's the sound of the third chakra, which rules the fire element.

9. Remember that fire during the day when you feel sluggish or dull.

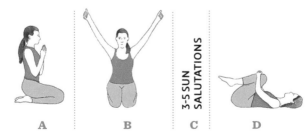

A   B   3-5 SUN SALUTATIONS   C   D

1. Start seated, cross-legged or sitting on a block. **A**

2. Rub your palms together gently.

3. Open your arms really wide, squeezing your shoulder blades together and opening your hands wide **B**, then cross your arms over your chest and give yourself a hug. **C**

4. Open your arms back out, and bring them back in, changing the crossing. Stay with this for two minutes or so.

5. Stand up and do three rounds of Sun Salutations (see page 45).

6. Finish by lying on your back in Reclining Goddess pose, feet together, knees apart falling out to the sides, a pillow under each knee. **E**

7. Place your hands gently on your belly and take 5 to 10 long breaths.

8. Finish sitting up, hands to your heart in prayer, and chant "hammmmm" one time. It's the sound of the fourth chakra, which rules the air element. **F**

9. Remember to breathe deeply during those times in your days when you may be feeling frustrated or judgmental.

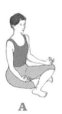
A

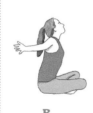
B

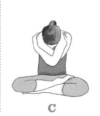
C

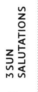

3 SUN SALUTATIONS

D

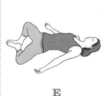
E

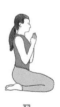
F

1. Start seated cross-legged or sitting on a block. **A**

2. Lightly place your right fingertips on the ground next to you, and let your left hand rest, palm down, on your left thigh. If you're sitting too high to get your hand down comfortably, put a yoga block or a firm pillow under your fingertips. This mudra is called Bhumisparsha mudra. *Bhu* means "earth" and *sparsha* means "touch". Bhumisparsha mudra is the mudra of touching the earth and staying connected to the ground.

3. Take five deep, slow breaths.

4. Come onto your hands and knees, wrists under your shoulders, knees under your hips, and begin Cat-Cow breathing: On the inhalation, arch your spine and look up into Cow, and on the exhalation, round your spine and press the ground away for Cat. Do this three to five times. **B, C**

5. Press back into Child's pose, hips to heels, forehead on the ground. **D**

6. Stay for another three breaths there, then come back onto your hands and knees. **B**

7. Tuck your toes under, and lift your hips up and back into Downward Facing Dog **E**. Stay for three breaths, then slowly walk forward to the top of your mat, coming into a Standing Forward Bend **F** with your feet about a fist's distance apart and your knees slightly bent. Slowly roll up, stacking the spine, keeping your knees bent until your head is upright.

8. Do two rounds of Sun Salutations (see page 46).

9. When you're done, lie down on your back in Savasana **H** and rest for three minutes, then bring your knees to your chest, roll over to one side, come up to sit, and bring your hands to your heart in prayer **I**. Chant "lammmmm" one time. It's the sound for the first chakra, which rules the earth element.

10. Remember that stability for those times in your day you feel spacey or anxious.

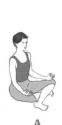
A

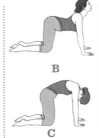
B
C

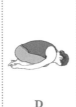
D

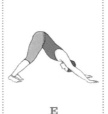
E

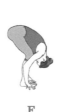
F

2 SUN SALUTATIONS G

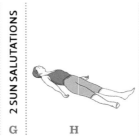
H

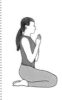
I

Kapha Variation

1. Start at the front of your mat in Tadasana (Mountain pose).

2. Inhale arms up, and exhale deeply bending your knees, coming into Utkatasana (Chair pose).

3. Inhale, and then exhale to fold forward into Uttanasana (Standing Forward Bend).

4. Inhale coming onto fingertips, lengthen spine, and look forward.

5. Exhale, plant palms, bend knees, and hop back into Chaturanga Dandasana (Four-Limbed Staff pose) or step back into Downward Facing Dog.

6. From Chaturanga, inhale Upward Facing Dog, exhale Downward Facing Dog.

7. Inhale step the right foot forward, exhale spin the back heel down.

8. Inhale up Warrior 1, exhale Chaturanga Dandasana.

9. Inhale Upward Facing Dog, exhale Downward Facing Dog.

10. Repeat left side.

11. Take five breaths in Downward Facing Dog.

12. Inhale look forward, exhale deeply bend knees and, with breath held out, hop or step forward.

13. Inhale onto fingertips and lengthen spine, exhale fold forward into Uttanasana.

14. Inhale Utkatasana, exhale Tadasana.

15. Repeat three to five times.

Pitta Variation

1. Start at the front of your mat in Tadasana.

2. Bring your hands together in Anjali mudra (Prayer Hands) at your heart.

3. Inhale hook your thumbs, soften your knees, and swing your arms forward, up, and slightly lean back, lifting the chest and looking up at hands, exhale fold forward into Uttanasana.

4. Inhale step the right foot back into a lunge, exhale Downward Facing Dog.

5. Inhale out to Plank pose, exhale lower to the ground or Chaturanga Dandasana.

6. Inhale up into Cobra or Upward Facing Dog, exhale Downward Facing Dog.

7. Inhale lift the right leg up, exhale step forward into a lunge.

8. Inhale left foot meets the right at the front of your mat, exhale fold forward into Uttanasana.

9. Inhale come up and stretch the arms up over your head, exhale hands to heart in Anjali mudra.

10. Repeat left side.

11. Repeat each side three times.

Vata Variation

1. Start at the front of your mat in a wide-legged Tadasana, feet as wide as shoulders.

2. Inhale stretch the arms up, join the palms above your head, and look up, exhale fold forward into Uttanasana.

3. Inhale step the right foot back into a lunge, exhale Downward Facing Dog.

4. Inhale rolling out to Plank pose as fluidly as possible, exhale lower to the ground or Chaturanga Dandasana.

5. Inhale Cobra or Upward Facing Dog, exhale Downward Facing Dog.

6. Inhale lift the right leg up, exhale step the right foot to the pinky side of the right hand, coming into a wide lunge.

7. Inhale, lift the right arm up, coming into a lunge twist, exhale place the right hand back down.

8. Inhale step the left foot wide of the left hand, exhale wide-footed forward bend.

9. Inhale lift up and stretch the arms over the head, exhale Tadasana.

10. Repeat other side.

11. Repeat for one more round.

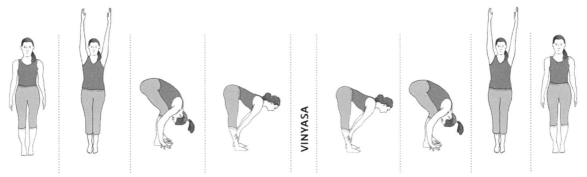

VINYASA

General Guidelines for Sun Salutations

QUICKER MORNING TIPS

Make your bed. It ritualizes the end of sleep, the beginning of a new day, and isn't it so much nicer to get into a well-made bed at night?

Light a stick of incense or put some essential oil in your diffuser. I like peppermint, wild orange, bergamot, grapefruit, or a combo of them for the morning.

Journal for a couple of minutes. Just stream of consciousness. This clears your head for what the day holds.

Nighttime Rituals

It's so easy to just come home after a long workday, heat something up, scarf it down, watch the latest show, and pass out. No wonder it seems like the days run into each other! Let's move into some simple ways to wind down and close out your days with relaxation and reflection.

- **Before prepping dinner, prep yourself.** Wash your hands and face well, and take off any rings, bracelets, or watches. If you have long hair, tie it back so it doesn't get in your face. If you have left mail or papers on the counter, clear them first so you have a clean space to work with. It doesn't need to be a big overhaul; just give yourself a space free of clutter.

- **Moon bathe.** This is one of my favorite Ayurvedic rituals. Think about it—we sunbathe, and that adds more heat to the body. Give yourself 20 minutes (or more!) relaxing outside under a full moon and pacify excess Pitta. If the full moon falls on a Monday (Moonday), it's even more potent. Put on some white or pale gray natural-fiber clothing, find a soft patch of ground (or a lounge chair on a rooftop), and let yourself take in the cooling gaze of Mama Moon. Bonus tip: If you're someone who is into mantra, the moon mantra is *"Om cham chandraya namaha,"* which means "I bow to the power of the Moon."

- **Give your feet some love!** When Vata or Pitta is high, insomnia can be an issue. You know proper sleep is essential for all the functions of your body to perform well. Maybe you can't get to sleep, or maybe you wake up in the middle of the night (usually around 2:30 to 3:00 a.m., right after Pitta time is over and Vata time has begun; airy Vata makes the Pitta fire flare up). Either situation will benefit from a bit of self-reflexology. Physically, our feet correspond with our first chakra, which is associated with the element of earth. Foot massage is so grounding. If your skin is very dry, use a palmful of organic sesame oil (I keep mine on my nightstand). And if it's not, use coconut oil. Add a few drops of cedarwood, lavender, or clary sage essential oil, and rub your palms together. Take a deep sniff, and then get to work! Rub the oil into the soles of your feet, the tops, your toes, around the ankles, and up to the calves. If the oil doesn't absorb instantly, put on some light cotton socks. Lie back down and close your eyes. Bonus tip: Rub a few drops of the same oil into the crown of your head for extra "weight."

Carve out five minutes to meditate. There are great guided meditations online. Find one for relaxation, set yourself up in a comfortable seat, let your eyes close, observe your breath, and follow instructions.

Do one restorative yoga pose for 5 to 10 minutes. Here are three options—pick one.

- ◆ Legs up the wall, lying on your back.

- ◆ Reclining Goddess pose, pillow under head and under each knee. Lie on your back with a pillow under your head. Bring your feet to the ground with your knees bent. Let your knees drop out to the sides, keeping the soles of your feet together (see page 43, E).

- ◆ Restorative Child's pose with a stack of pillows under your belly and a blanket under your knees and feet. Come onto your hands and knees with a stack of three pillows nearby. Bring your hips to your heels as you reach for the pillows. Put them under your belly and release your arms on either side of the pillows or gently slide your hands under the pillows if that feels nice to you. You can turn your head to one side for two minutes or so, then change sides (see page 44, D).

Once you're in bed, pick the top three favorite moments of your day and replay them in your mind. Contemplate why you chose those moments: Was it something you learned, something you taught, something that made your heart melt?

Bathing Rituals

Anytime you have access to a bathtub, clear some time for a bath. It is so soothing for the nervous system! Here's a basic recipe for bath salts that can be adjusted for the season.

1 cup Epsom salts

¼ cup baking soda

¼ cup Himalayan salt

Seasonal essential oils

1. Get a glass jar with a lid that holds 2 cups.
2. Pour in the Epsom salts, baking soda, and Himalayan salt.
3. Add your chosen essential oils, and shake well.
4. Let the salts sit overnight if possible.
5. When you run your bath, add ½ cup to your bathwater. Ahhhh . . .

- ♦ **Kapha Season** Add the following essential oils: 2 drops wild orange, 2 drops grapefruit, 2 drops rosemary, and 2 drops peppermint.
- ♦ **Pitta Season** Add the following essential oils: 2 drops jasmine (the good stuff is pricey, so if you don't want to spend the money, substitute ylang ylang oil), 4 drops lavender, and 2 drops clary sage.
- ♦ **Vata Season** Add the following essential oils: 2 drops geranium, 4 drops lavender, 2 drops lemongrass, and 2 drops cedarwood.

QUICKER BATHING TIP

No bathtub? No worries! Take the same essential oil recipes, add them to a lava stone, and place it in the corner of your shower.

Seasonal Rituals

In Ayurveda, we call this *ritucharya,* or seasonal routines. Here are some suggestions regarding appropriate actions for each season.

KAPHA SEASON

This is the time of year to cleanse, detox, and refresh!

- ♦ **Cleanse.** Try a three-day kichadi cleanse (see page 56).
- ♦ **Spring clean.** It doesn't have to be an all-day thing. Start small. Start with your drawers. If that feels too overwhelming, start with one drawer. My go-to is my T-shirt drawer. Throw out the T-shirts that have rips or stains, or those that have become faded beyond recognition (well, you can keep one oversized and sentimental comfort shirt. But just one!). Fold your T-shirts neatly, and stack them by color. Put a couple of drops of eucalyptus, lavender, or rosemary essential oil on a cotton ball, and place it in the corner of the drawer.
- ♦ **Care for your hair and skin.** Cut your hair, trim your nails, and use a body brush or loofah to slough off tired winter skin and promote circulation.

PITTA SEASON

This is the time of year for celebration and connection.

- ◆ **Have a picnic.** When was the last time you had one? You don't need the perfect beach or forest. Find a park, a terrace, or a rooftop on a beautiful warm day, and invite some friends for a festive weekend lunch.
- ◆ **Do charity work.** Charity work, while good all year, is especially important in Pitta season, because it connects us to the heart. Chop veggies for a soup kitchen, make brownies for a bake sale for your kid's soccer team, or devote some time to making phone calls for a specific charity that resonates with you.
- ◆ **Sing!** It's so heart opening! Join a choir, go to a concert where you know all the words to all the songs, or just blast some music while you shower and let yourself wail. My client Traci says, "You cannot tell me I'm not Mary J. Blige every morning!"

VATA SEASON

This is the time of year for, as I like to say, nesting and resting.

- ◆ **Invite a small group of friends over for a potluck.** Make a big batch of yummy soup, and have someone bring the appetizer, someone else the side dish, someone else the beverage, someone else the dessert. Stretch out the meal and the evening with a fun movie or a silly game. This gets us out of isolation mode.
- ◆ **Change your comforter.** Swap out the light color and weight for something a little darker and heavier for cozy nights. The weight of the blanket is very good for the lightness of Vata.

♦ **Get a massage.** Specifically, get into *abhyanga*, also known as Ayurvedic oil massage. Get some sesame oil, and add a few drops of essential oils to it. For Vata season, think warming. I like to take one cup of base oil, put it in a glass jar (this is important, as essential oils leach chemicals from plastic), and add two drops of cinnamon, two drops of cedarwood, four drops of lavender, and two drops of wild orange. Post-shower, take a handful and give yourself a rubdown. Make some extra circles around your joints: ankles, knees, hips, shoulders, elbows, and wrists. If you're like me, it will sink in quickly. If it doesn't, jump back in the shower and do a "turnaround" (i.e., set the water to warm, and turn around under it to get the barest minimum of a rinse, then towel off lightly).

Living Consciously

Ritualizing our days is so fulfilling! Infuse your life with meaning, and it will be easier to stay present. With presence and awareness, you feel as if you are cocreating your life instead of your life just happening to you. Trust the process. Small shifts in diet, routines, and lifestyle add up. If you miss a day here and there, just get right back into it as soon as you're able. It never needs to be an all-or-nothing situation. Let your approach be loving and patient.

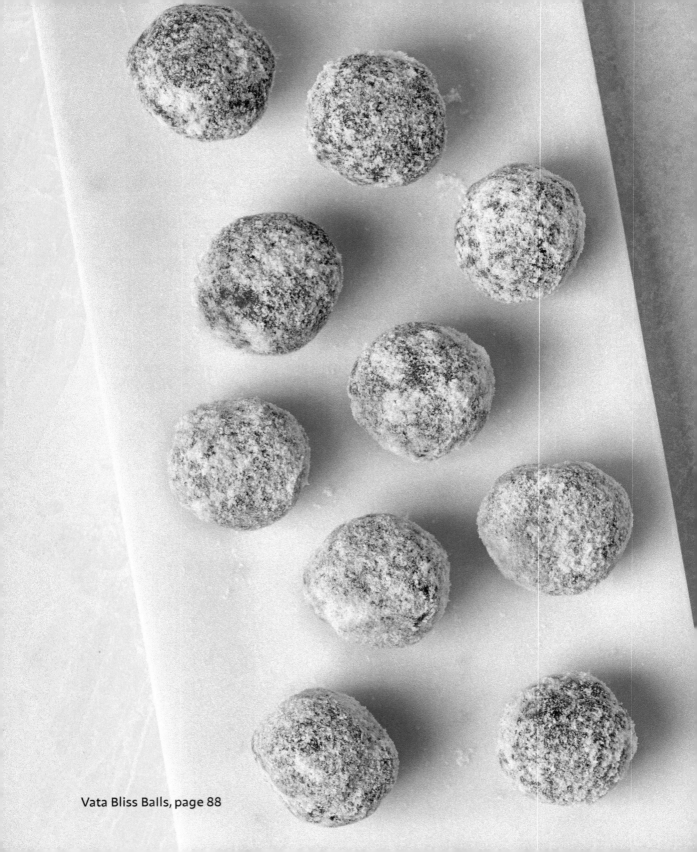

Vata Bliss Balls, page 88

4
RECIPES FOR HEALING AND DETOX

This chapter will include some ideas for breakfast, lunch, dinner, snacks, and tonics. Keep in mind that Ayurvedic theory stresses the importance of how we eat our meals, not just what is in our bowls. Try to eat all of your meals without rush, in a calm and peaceful environment. Stay off electronics while you're eating, chew your food well, don't drink too much liquid while you're eating, and always offer a prayer of gratitude for the opportunity to nourish yourself well. For your convenience, I have included labels with each recipe that let you know if the recipe is vegan, vegetarian, and/or gluten-free. You'll notice that many recipes are easy to adapt to your diet, even if they are not labeled as such. As always, be sure to carefully inspect packaging to ensure foods, particularly oats, were processed in a completely gluten-free facility before using them.

About the Recipes...

- **Kichadi** An Ayurvedic staple dish. You might see it spelled kichari, kitchari, or kchri—it's all the same thing. It's a grain-and-bean combination packed with digestive spices.

- **Breakfast** Each dosha has different needs for breakfast. I find this is the time of day where most of my clients really want something fast, simple, and nourishing.

- **Spice It Up!** Herbs and spices support digestion, immunity, and cleansing and can take your food from blah to wow in one sprinkle. We blend them for optimal benefits. These blends are called *masalas* and can be made ahead of time in a big batch and added to any dish. These masala recipes make enough to last about a month. When you are done making the masala, put it in an airtight glass jar away from heat.

- **Blank-Canvas Dishes** These are some of my customizable Blank-Canvas Dishes (affectionately known as "BCDs") to add masalas to and play with in the kitchen.

- **Simple Soups** Soups are easy to prepare, healthy, and easily reheated. As mentioned, Ayurveda does not recommend making leftovers a habit, but if choosing between takeout or your own food reheated, go for your own every time.

- **A Burger for Everyone!** Who doesn't love a good veggie burger? If you're going for low-carb, have the burger over a plate of veggies. Gluten-free? Doesn't *everything* taste better in a taco? Get some organic corn tortillas, either soft (Pitta and Vata) or crunchy (Kapha).

- **Condiments** I recruited some friends to share their condiment recipes. These can be used anytime you need a hit of extra flavor and specialness for an otherwise simple dish.

- **Snacks** Sometimes our day stretches on longer than we planned, and we need a little something to feed the digestive fire.

- **Tonics** For when you need something grounding, there are milk-based tonics.

THE HEALING RECIPES

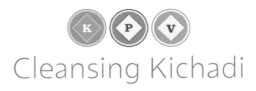

Cleansing Kichadi

GLUTEN-FREE / VEGAN

PREP TIME: 20 MINUTES | COOK TIME: 55 MINUTES | SERVES 2

Here's the traditional kichadi recipe, appropriate for all doshas. It has mung dal and white basmati rice, as white rice is easier to digest than brown rice. It's fun to experiment by switching out the rice for quinoa or trying a new kind of rice. You can also add garnishes such as coconut flakes, chopped cilantro or parsley, a drizzle of ghee or coconut oil, or even hemp seeds.

1 tablespoon coconut oil (Pitta), ghee or sesame oil (Vata), or sunflower oil (Kapha)

1 teaspoon black mustard seeds

1 teaspoon cumin seeds

½ teaspoon fennel seeds

½ teaspoon fenugreek seeds, ground cinnamon (in winter), or Dosha Masala (pages 64–66)

1 dried bay leaf

1 teaspoon ground turmeric

1 teaspoon freshly ground black pepper

½ teaspoon ground cumin

½ teaspoon ground coriander

½ cup yellow mung dal beans, rinsed well

6 cups water

2 green cardamom pods

1 whole clove

1 to 3 cups chopped vegetables appropriate for your dosha (see table on page 94)

½ cup white basmati rice

Chopped fresh cilantro, for garnish

1. In a large stockpot over medium heat, heat the oil. Add the black mustard, cumin seeds, fennel, and fenugreek, and toast until the mustard seeds pop.

2. Add the bay leaf, turmeric, black pepper, cumin, and coriander, and mix together.

3. Stir in the mung dal beans.

4. Add the water, cardamom pods, clove, and chopped vegetables. Bring to a boil, then lower the heat to medium-low. Simmer for 30 minutes, then add the rice and cook for another 20 minutes, or until the beans and rice are soft and the kichadi has a soupy consistency.

5. Garnish with cilantro and serve.

Erleichda (Lighten Up!) Kichadi

GLUTEN-FREE / VEGAN
PREP TIME: 15 MINUTES, PLUS OVERNIGHT TO SOAK
COOK TIME: 1 HOUR 35 MINUTES | SERVES 4

This kichadi is full of delicious heating spices for Kapha digestion. If you have never tried millet, see if you can get your hands on some! It's delicious, warming, and slightly drying. Chickpeas have the astringent taste, which is beneficial for excess Kapha.

½ cup dried chickpeas

10 cups water, divided

1 to 2 tablespoons peeled and minced fresh ginger

½ teaspoon ground cinnamon

¼ teaspoon whole cloves

1 cup millet or basmati rice

4 dried bay leaves

2 tablespoons extra-virgin olive oil

¼ teaspoon sea salt

Kapha Masala, for sprinkling (page 64; optional)

1. Soak the chickpeas overnight, then drain.

2. In a large stockpot over medium-high heat, combine the soaked chickpeas and 6 cups of water. Bring to a boil, then lower the heat to medium-low and simmer, uncovered, for 10 minutes, skimming any foam off the surface. Drain the chickpeas, return them to the pot, and add the remaining 4 cups of water. Return to a boil over medium-high heat.

3. Add the ginger, cinnamon, and cloves. Lower the heat to medium-low, and simmer for 1 hour.

4. Add the millet, bay leaves, olive oil, and salt to the chickpea mixture, and stir.

5. Cover, lower the heat to low, and cook for 20 to 25 minutes, until the chickpeas are soft enough to mush with a spoon.

6. Top with a sprinkle of masala (if using), and serve.

Cool-It-Down Kichadi

GLUTEN-FREE / VEGETARIAN

PREP TIME: 15 MINUTES, PLUS 3 HOURS TO SOAK | COOK TIME: 40 MINUTES | SERVES 4

The bitterness of cilantro makes it one of the best herbs for cooling the Pitta fire, and coconut adds a cooling sweetness to this dish.

½ cup mung dal beans, rinsed well

1 (1-inch) piece fresh ginger, peeled and chopped

⅓ cup dried unsweetened coconut flakes

⅓ cup chopped fresh cilantro

6½ cups water, divided

2 tablespoons ghee or coconut oil

½ teaspoon ground turmeric

¼ teaspoon sea salt

1 cup basmati rice, rinsed well

Pitta Masala, for sprinkling (page 65, optional)

1. Soak the mung dal beans for 3 hours, then drain and set aside.

2. In a high-speed blender or food processor, combine the ginger, coconut, cilantro, and ½ cup of water, and blend well.

3. In a large saucepan over medium heat, combine the ghee, the cilantro mixture, turmeric, and salt. Stir well, and bring to a boil.

4. Mix in the soaked mung dal beans and the remaining 6 cups of water. Return to a boil.

5. Add the rice, and stir well. Boil, uncovered, for 5 minutes. Then partially cover, lower the heat to medium-low, and simmer for 25 to 30 minutes, until the beans and rice are soft.

6. Top with a sprinkle of masala (if using), and serve.

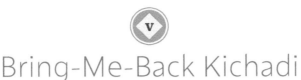

Bring-Me-Back Kichadi

GLUTEN-FREE / VEGETARIAN
PREP TIME: 20 MINUTES, PLUS 3 HOURS TO SOAK
COOK TIME: 1 HOUR 15 MINUTES | SERVES 4 TO 6

The spices in this kichadi are so medicinal for Vata digestion! Notice the good fats in the sesame oil or ghee—so helpful for combating dryness. Sweet potatoes are grounding, and they add a small amount of sodium and slow-absorbing carbohydrates, which is great for boosting stamina.

1 cup split mung beans, rinsed well in cold water

1 cup brown basmati rice, rinsed well

1 (1½-inch) piece fresh ginger, peeled and grated

½ cup fresh cilantro leaves

2 tablespoons shredded fresh or dried unsweetened coconut

1 teaspoon ground turmeric

3 tablespoons ghee or sesame oil

11 whole black peppercorns or ½ teaspoon freshly ground black pepper

Seeds from 8 green cardamom pods

8 whole cloves

3 dried bay leaves

1 (3-inch) cinnamon stick

1 to 2 large sweet potatoes, cubed

1 teaspoon sea salt

Vata Masala, for sprinkling (page 66, optional)

1. Soak the split mung beans for 3 hours, then drain and set aside. Soak the rice while the kichadi is cooking.

2. In a high-speed blender or food processor, combine the ginger, cilantro, coconut, and turmeric with enough water to blend easily. Blend well, and set aside.

3. In a large stockpot over medium heat, heat the ghee. Add the black peppercorns, cardamom, cloves, bay leaves, and cinnamon stick, and sauté for 2 to 3 minutes.

4. Add the ginger-turmeric mixture, and sauté for 2 to 3 more minutes, until lightly cooked.

5. Add the soaked split mung beans and sweet potatoes, and sauté for 3 to 4 minutes.

6. Add water to cover by 3 to 5 inches, and bring to a boil over medium-high heat. Lower the heat to medium-low, and simmer for 35 to 45 minutes, or until the split mung beans are completely broken down.

7. Add the rice, and cook for another 20 minutes, until the rice is soft and mushy. Add more water as needed to get a soupy consistency. Add the salt, and give the kichadi a final good stir.

8. Top with a sprinkle of masala (if using), and serve.

Kapha Breakfasts

Kapha, you need a light, refreshing breakfast. Try the Erleichda (Lighten Up!) Kichadi recipe (see page 58) or one of these ideas.

▪ **Chickpea pancakes.** These are so yummy. When I was in northern India, my hostess used to make these every morning as a breakfast option. Chickpea flour, or besan, can be found online or in an Indian market. It's gluten-free, contains protein, and is incredibly versatile.

1. Mix 1 cup of chickpea flour with ½ teaspoon of sea salt and enough water to make a batter.
2. If you have cilantro or chives on hand, chop some up and add them to the batter.
3. Heat a well-seasoned cast iron or stainless steel pan over medium heat, lightly grease with olive oil, and pour out about ¼ cup of the batter. Don't touch! Allow the batter to cook for 3 minutes without flipping, then flip and cook on the other side for another 3 minutes. Transfer the pancake to a plate, and top with a drizzle of raw organic honey.

▪ **Grapefruit.** This is light and good for your metabolism. Peel a grapefruit, cut it into pieces, and sprinkle it with some ground cinnamon. Easy-peasy.

▪ **Tofu scramble.** This comes together so quickly!

1. Crumble about ⅓ of a block of extra-firm tofu.
2. Mix it with 1 tablespoon of diced onion, 1 tablespoon of diced carrot, and ¼ cup finely chopped kale.
3. Heat a well-seasoned cast iron or stainless steel pan over medium heat, and add 1 teaspoon of sunflower oil. Add the tofu-vegetable mixture, a pinch each of ground turmeric and freshly ground black pepper, and 1 tablespoon of liquid aminos or soy sauce.
4. Cook for 5 minutes, add a dash of hot sauce, and serve.

Pitta Breakfasts

Pitta, you need a breakfast that is satisfying without being too heavy. Again, the Cool-It-Down Kichadi recipe (see page 59) would work if you love a savory breakfast. Otherwise, here are some ideas for you.

- **Smoothie.** A smoothie is a nice breakfast for Pitta types. Here's a base—feel free to embellish. Blend together 1 banana, 1 cup of coconut water, a pinch ground cardamom, and a big squeeze of lime juice. Then try optional add-ins such as frozen or fresh blueberries, coconut flakes, ½ of a small avocado (which makes it almost pudding-like), and fresh mint.

- **Whole-grain toast.** Add a smear of coconut butter, and this is your quick, easy go-to.

- **Overnight oats.** Combine ½ cup of oats, 1 cup of almond or coconut milk, a few almonds, a pinch of ground cardamom, and some goji berries or 1 chopped date in a jar, and leave in the fridge overnight.

Vata Breakfasts

Vata, you need a grounding breakfast, and warm is usually a better fit than cold. Skip the cold, raw smoothie! The Bring-Me-Back Kichadi (see page 60) is always an option, or I often recommend the following.

- **Warming breakfast cereal.** This is made of cooked grains (such as oatmeal, quinoa, or basmati rice) with a pinch of ground cinnamon; almond, coconut, or dairy milk; and a drizzle of maple syrup. Then try optional add-ins such as a sprinkle of chia seeds, hemp hearts, chopped almonds, and coconut flakes, and a spoonful of protein powder.

- **Quick sandwich.** Smear 1 to 2 slices of hearty whole-grain bread with almond butter.

- **Yogurt.** This can be dairy or nondairy yogurt (I like cashew) with 1 teaspoon each of any of the optional add-ins from the warming cereal. Note that this is best for warmer weather.

ABOUT ANJALIS

Traditional Ayurveda uses measurements called *anjalis*. I love that because the Anjali mudra is hands pressed together at the heart, or what we think of as Prayer Hands. Your anjali is specific to you. One anjali is both hands cupped together like a bowl. One-half anjali is one handful, and so on. During my first Ayurvedic training, that was all we used—no cups or teaspoons. Every recipe was "1 anjali" or a "3-finger pinch" or a "5-finger pinch." So, while we were all cooking the same thing, the results were slightly different for everyone. I adore this practice because it makes cooking much more personalized.

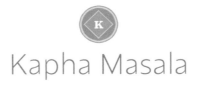

Kapha Masala

GLUTEN-FREE / VEGAN

**COOK TIME: 15 TO 30 MINUTES, DEPENDING ON WHETHER
YOU USE A MORTAR AND PESTLE | MAKES 1½ CUPS**

This masala has a kick to it! The pungency of the spices gives you a good boost when you're feeling low energy. Remember that pungent is considered too heating for Pitta and Vata types. If you don't have a mortar and pestle, use a coffee grinder.

¼ anjali garlic powder

½ anjali ground ginger

5-finger pinch ground turmeric

5-finger pinch paprika

½ anjali cumin seeds

¼ anjali black mustard seeds

3-finger pinch whole black peppercorns

---

1. In a big bowl, combine the garlic, ginger, turmeric, and paprika.

2. In a small, cast iron or stainless steel pan over medium heat, dry roast the cumin, stirring gently, for a few minutes, until the seeds are slightly browned and fragrant. Carefully spoon them into a large, stone mortar. Using the pestle, grind the cumin to a powder. Add the ground cumin to the garlic-spice mixture.

3. Add the black mustard seeds to the pan, still over medium heat. Be careful—they pop! Step back and give them a good stir, until the seeds change color from black to gray. Remove them from the heat. Carefully spoon them into a large stone mortar. Using the pestle, grind the black mustard seeds to a powder. Add the ground black mustard to the garlic-spice mixture.

4. Add the black peppercorns to the pan, still over medium heat. Dry roast them, stirring gently, until they are fragrant. Carefully spoon them into a large, stone mortar. Using the pestle, grind the black peppercorns to a powder. Add the ground black pepper to the garlic-spice mixture.

5. Transfer the masala to a glass jar with a lid, secure the lid, and give it a vigorous shake to blend.

6. To retain freshness, store away from light and heat for up to 1 month.

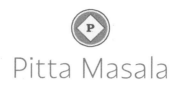

Pitta Masala

GLUTEN-FREE / VEGAN

**COOK TIME: 15 TO 30 MINUTES, DEPENDING ON WHETHER YOU
USE A MORTAR AND PESTLE | MAKES ABOUT 2 CUPS**

This masala is great for those with Pitta as their main constitution. It can also work for other doshas in the summer. This recipe makes a lot, so share generously! If you don't have a mortar and pestle, use a coffee grinder.

5-finger pinch ground turmeric

3-finger pinch saffron

3-finger pinch coconut sugar (optional)

1 anjali coriander seeds

½ anjali cumin seeds

¼ anjali fennel seeds

¼ anjali whole white peppercorns

---

1. In a small bowl, combine the turmeric, saffron, and coconut sugar (if using), and set aside.

2. In a small, cast iron or stainless steel pan over medium heat, dry roast the coriander seeds, stirring gently, for a few minutes, until the seeds are fragrant. Carefully spoon them into a large, stone mortar. Using the pestle, grind the coriander seeds to a powder. Transfer the ground coriander to a glass jar with a lid.

3. Repeat this dry roasting and grinding process with the cumin seeds, fennel seeds, and white peppercorns.

4. Add the turmeric mixture to the jar, secure with the lid, and give it a vigorous shake to blend.

5. To retain freshness, store away from light and heat for up to 1 month.

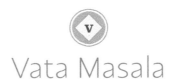

Vata Masala

GLUTEN-FREE / VEGAN

**COOK TIME: 15 TO 30 MINUTES, DEPENDING ON WHETHER
YOU USE A MORTAR AND PESTLE | MAKES 1 CUP**

This masala is spicy without being pungent, and the sesame seeds release a bit of oil, which adds some good fats. If you don't have a mortar and pestle, use a coffee grinder.

½ anjali sesame seeds

½ anjali cumin seeds

¼ anjali yellow mustard seeds

5-finger pinch coriander seeds

5-finger pinch whole cloves

1 (3-inch) cinnamon stick

1. In a small cast iron or stainless steel pan over medium heat, dry roast the sesame seeds, stirring gently, for a few minutes, until they are fragrant. Transfer them to a medium bowl, and set aside.

2. Repeat this dry roasting process with the cumin seeds, yellow mustard seeds, coriander seeds, cloves, and cinnamon stick.

3. Then, one spoonful at a time, transfer the spice mixture to a large, stone mortar. Using the pestle, grind the spices to a powder. The cinnamon will take some work, so dig in with all you have!

4. Transfer the masala to a glass jar with a lid, secure the lid, and give it a vigorous shake to blend.

5. To retain freshness, store away from light and heat for up to 1 month.

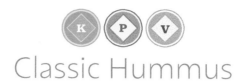

Classic Hummus

GLUTEN-FREE / VEGAN
PREP TIME: 10 MINUTES | SERVES 4

I strongly recommend you make a batch of this and keep it in the refrigerator for those nights you are too tired to cook. It's kind of a clichéd dish for us yoga teachers, but I always say clichés become clichés for a reason. I once invited some yoga friends to a picnic and told everyone to bring something, and we ended up with six different kinds of hummus and some raspberry-lime seltzer. We were all fine with it.

1 (15-ounce) can chickpeas, drained and rinsed, or 1½ cups cooked dried chickpeas

1 to 2 tablespoons tahini

Juice of ½ lemon, plus more if needed

1 tablespoon extra-virgin olive oil (omit for Kapha)

1 garlic clove, peeled and raw or roasted (use raw for Kapha, use roasted for Vata, and omit for Pitta)

1 teaspoon masala of choice (page 64–66) or ½ teaspoon ground cumin, plus more if needed

Masala of choice or paprika, for garnish

Sea salt

¼ cup water (if needed)

1. In a high-speed blender or food processor, combine the chickpeas, tahini, lemon juice, olive oil, garlic, and masala.

2. Purée until the mixture forms a paste. Add the water as needed, then taste and season with salt. Add additional lemon juice and spices as needed.

3. Sprinkle with a little extra masala, and serve.

Sweeten-Me-Up Hummus

GLUTEN-FREE / VEGAN
PREP TIME: 10 MINUTES | SERVES 4

This hummus is more suitable for Vata people or as a treat for Pitta and Kapha constitutions in Vata season. It uses pinto beans, which are usually a no-no for Vata (see the food list on page 94), but the addition of spices and sweet potato, as well as the blending, make it more appropriate. If you don't have any Vata Masala, substitute ½ teaspoon each of ground cumin and cinnamon.

1 (15-ounce) can pinto beans, drained and rinsed

1 small sweet potato, roasted

1 tablespoon coconut oil

1 tablespoon apple cider vinegar, plus more if needed

1 tablespoon Vata Masala (page 66), plus more for garnish

5-finger pinch sea salt, plus more if needed

¼ cup water (if needed)

1. In a high-speed blender or food processor, combine the beans, sweet potato, coconut oil, vinegar, masala, and salt.

2. Purée until the mixture forms a paste. Add the water as needed, then taste and adjust the vinegar, salt, and spices as necessary.

3. Sprinkle with a little extra masala, and serve.

HUMMUS TRANSPORT

There are so many ways to enjoy your hummus! You can keep it gluten-free and dosha-appropriate. Here are some ideas to get you started.

♦ **Kapha**—Raw carrot and celery sticks, raw red or daikon radishes, rice crackers or rice cakes, or a bowl of cooked millet or white potato.

♦ **Pitta**—Raw cucumber and celery sticks, pita bread, rice crackers or rice cakes, a bowl of cooked rice, or white or sweet potato.

♦ **Vata**—Roasted veggies (sweet potato, carrots, winter squash, turnips, beets), pita bread, or a bowl of cooked rice or quinoa.

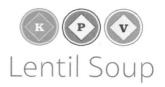

Lentil Soup

GLUTEN-FREE / VEGAN

PREP TIME: 10 MINUTES | COOK TIME: 50 MINUTES | SERVES 4

We can go down the list: Easy, check. Delicious, check. Inexpensive, check. Quick, check. Again, this is one to make a pot of and stretch it for two dinners and two lunches—or make a big pot and invite friends over. For the veggie broth, read the label; some of them are too high in salt and preservatives.

2 to 3 tablespoons extra-virgin olive oil (2 for Kapha and Pitta, 3 for Vata)

4 garlic cloves, minced (omit for Pitta)

2 carrots, peeled and diced

1 medium onion, diced

1 tablespoon masala of choice (pages 64–66), plus more for serving

1 (28-ounce) can diced tomatoes, lightly drained

4 cups vegetable broth

2 cups water

1 cup brown or green lentils, rinsed well

1 cup chopped, stemmed fresh kale or arugula

Juice of ½ lemon

1 teaspoon sea salt

1. In a large stockpot over medium heat, heat the olive oil for 2 minutes. Add the garlic, carrots, and onion. Cook for 5 minutes, gently stirring every minute or so.

2. Add the masala and cook, stirring frequently, for 1 minute. Then add the tomatoes and cook, stirring gently, for 3 minutes.

3. Add the broth, water, and lentils. Bring to a boil, then lower the heat to medium-low. Partially cover, and simmer for 25 to 30 minutes.

4. Add the kale, and simmer for another 5 minutes.

5. Remove the pot from the heat, and add the lemon juice and salt. Give the soup a big stir.

6. Serve, and pass a bowl of the masala around.

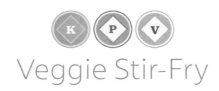

Veggie Stir-Fry

GLUTEN-FREE / VEGETARIAN

PREP TIME: 15 MINUTES | COOK TIME: 10 TO 20 MINUTES | SERVES 2 TO 4

Truth be told, I make a variation of this blank canvas dish (BCD) at least five times a week. You can just swap out the oil, spices, or veggies and totally change the taste. I have included a table that lists vegetables from slowest cooking time to quickest. You don't want to cook everything all at once, or you'll end up with overcooked vegetables. Try to choose one to two vegetables from each group, starting with the slowest-cooking vegetables and "layering" in more as you go. You can put this stir-fry over a grain bowl, add a protein, and voila! You're good to go for lunch or dinner. See the food lists on page 94 for appropriate vegetables, grains, and cooking oils. If you're not using any of the vegetables from one group, no worries—the stir-fry will still taste great!

---

2 tablespoons oil or ghee (see sidebar)

1 to 2 tablespoons spice blend (see sidebar) or masala of choice

3 cups chopped vegetables of choice

Sea salt

---

1. In a large skillet over medium heat, heat the oil until hot. Add the spice blend.

2. Add the slowest-cooking vegetables according to the table, making sure not to crowd the pan. If you put too many veggies in all at once, they release too much water and everything starts to steam instead of fry. Season to taste with salt. Cook for a couple of minutes without stirring. Then continue to cook, stirring occasionally and adding faster-cooking vegetables, until the chunky vegetables are tender and caramelized and the leafy vegetables are wilted but not limp. The whole process should take 10 to 20 minutes, depending on the vegetables.

3. Taste, add additional salt as needed, serve.

Slow	Medium	Fast
Mushrooms	Peppers	Spinach
Onions	Kale	Dandelion
Broccoli	Garlic	Baby arugula
Cauliflower	Tomatoes	Baby kale
Carrots	Okra	Swiss chard leaves
Brussels sprouts	Eggplant	Summer squash
Daikon radish	Broccoli rabe	Zucchini
Sweet potato	Collard greens	Herbs
White potato	Swiss chard stems	
Winter squash	String beans	

WANNA MAKE IT TASTE . . .

Here's a list of some traditional flavors found in a few cuisines. Of course, I'm not suggesting that this is an exact ingredient list. As with all regional cooking, there are hundreds of variations, but this should get you started in your experimenting with BCDs.

- **Italian-style.** Use olive oil, garlic, onion, tomato, basil, oregano, rosemary, Italian parsley, salt, and black pepper.

- **Thai-style.** Use coconut oil, garlic, onion, basil (Thai basil if you can find it), cilantro, coriander, cumin, coconut milk (this makes everything taste good), ginger, kaffir lime leaves (harder to find, but totally worth it) chiles, salt, and soy sauce.

- **Chinese-style.** Use toasted or regular sesame oil, garlic, chiles, onion, ginger, soy sauce, and Chinese five-spice powder (see resources on page 158).

- **Ethiopian-style.** Use olive oil, onion, garlic, chiles, paprika, cayenne, ginger, cumin, coriander, cardamom, fenugreek, cinnamon, nutmeg, allspice, and cloves or berbere (see resources on page 158).

- **Indian-style.** Use ghee or the oil most appropriate for your dosha. Use your masala! Or get some garam masala (see resources on page 158).

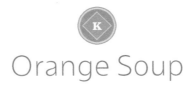

Orange Soup

GLUTEN-FREE / VEGAN

PREP TIME: 10 MINUTES | COOK TIME: 10 MINUTES | SERVES 4

Kapha soup recipes are full of flavor without making you feel heavy. In this recipe, the ginger and carrots add heat, and the celery has a slight diuretic quality, which is good for excess Kapha dampness in the body.

---

4 carrots, peeled

2 celery stalks

1 (2-inch) piece fresh ginger, peeled

1 tablespoon extra-virgin olive oil

½ teaspoon sea salt

5-finger pinch freshly ground black pepper

½ teaspoon Kapha Masala (page 64)

Chopped fresh cilantro, for garnish

---

1. In a high-speed blender, combine the carrots, celery, and ginger. Add enough water to cover them. Purée until the mixture is smooth. (If you have a small blender, do this step in two batches.)

2. Transfer the mixture to a large saucepan over medium heat. Add the olive oil, salt, black pepper, and masala. Cook, stirring occasionally, until heated through.

3. Garnish the soup with cilantro, and serve.

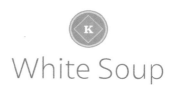

White Soup

GLUTEN-FREE / VEGAN
PREP TIME: 10 MINUTES | COOK TIME: 30 MINUTES | SERVES 4

Potatoes get a bad rap because they are often prepared with a lot of not-so-healthy add-ins. They show up on menus with heaps of butter, sour cream, cheese, and bacon, or they are fried and heavily salted. Any of these preparations can make you feel heavy and slow. Yet, white potatoes are recommended for Kapha types, as their *rasa*, or taste, is astringent. The astringent quality is light, dry, and cooling. This recipe is simple, nutritious, and full of flavor from the spices and leek. Fennel, cayenne, and black pepper increase agni and help burn away excess ama.

---

4 cups water

4 medium red potatoes, peeled and cubed

1 leek, rinsed well

2 cups cold water

2 tablespoons sunflower oil

1 tablespoon fennel seeds

1 teaspoon freshly ground black pepper or Kapha Masala (page 64)

½ teaspoon sea salt

5-finger pinch ground cayenne

---

1. In a large stockpot over medium-high heat, heat the water.

2. Add the potatoes, and bring to a boil. Cook for 10 minutes, until tender.

3. While the potatoes cook, chop the leek.

4. Drain the potatoes, reserving the water and setting it aside. Transfer the potatoes to a high-speed blender. Add the chopped leek and cold water. Purée until the mixture is smooth. (If you have a small blender, do this step in two batches.)

5. Transfer the potato-leek mixture back to the stockpot, and return to a boil over medium-high heat. Add the reserved water, sunflower oil, fennel, black pepper, salt, and cayenne. Lower the heat to medium-low, and simmer for 20 minutes.

6. Serve.

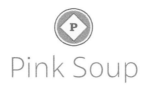

Pink Soup

GLUTEN-FREE / VEGAN
PREP TIME: 10 MINUTES | COOK TIME: 30 MINUTES | SERVES 4

Pitta-balancing soups are cooling and either slightly sweet or bitter. Cooked beets are sweeter than raw ones, which is better for Pitta digestion.

2 medium or 3 small beets, washed well and quartered

1½ cups water, plus more if needed

1 (1-inch) piece fresh ginger, peeled and grated

½ cup coconut flakes

3 tablespoons coconut oil

1 teaspoon Pitta Masala (page 65) or 5-finger pinch freshly ground black pepper

¼ teaspoon sea salt

Chopped fresh cilantro, for garnish

1. Combine the beets and water in a high-speed blender. Purée until the mixture is smooth.

2. Transfer the beet mixture to a stockpot over medium-high heat. Add the ginger, coconut flakes, coconut oil, masala, and salt, and bring to a boil.

3. Lower the heat to medium-low and simmer, partially covered, for 25 minutes. Add more water if the soup is too thick.

4. Garnish with cilantro and serve.

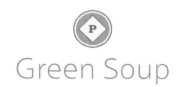

Green Soup

GLUTEN-FREE / VEGAN
PREP TIME: 15 MINUTES | SERVES 4

Cucumbers are one of the best Pitta-pacifying gifts we have from Mother Nature. Both mint and cilantro are cooling and good for Pitta digestion, and the small amount of ginger keeps the balance in check. The coconut garnish is optional, but so delicious!

2 cups fresh cilantro leaves

2 fresh mint leaves

1 (1-inch) piece fresh ginger, peeled

2 cups water

1 large cucumber, peeled and diced

Juice of ½ lime

1 tablespoon sunflower oil

¼ teaspoon sea salt

Coconut flakes or coconut yogurt, for garnish

1. In a high-speed blender, combine the cilantro, mint, and ginger. Add the water, and purée until the mixture is smooth. Strain the cilantro mixture, and return it to the blender.

2. Add the cucumber, lime juice, sunflower oil, and salt, blending to combine.

3. Garnish with coconut flakes, and serve immediately at room temperature.

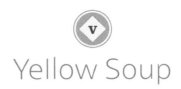

Yellow Soup

GLUTEN-FREE / VEGETARIAN
PREP TIME: 15 MINUTES | COOK TIME: 75 MINUTES | SERVES 4

Ah, Vata-balancing recipes! This is true comfort food—it's hearty and filling for a cold winter evening. Make up a batch and invite over a couple of lucky friends to share. This dish is also great for holiday parties.

1 (3-pound) butternut squash, halved lengthwise and seeded

1 teaspoon, extra-virgin olive oil, plus 1 tablespoon

1½ teaspoons sea salt, divided

Pinch freshly ground black pepper

1 to 2 tablespoons ghee or extra-virgin olive oil

1 large shallot or small sweet onion, chopped

4 garlic cloves, pressed or minced

4 cups vegetable broth

1 teaspoon maple syrup

½ teaspoon vanilla extract (optional)

¼ teaspoon ground nutmeg

Ghee or extra-virgin olive oil, for drizzling

1. Preheat the oven to 425°F. Place the squash on a roasting pan. Rub the cut side with 1 teaspoon of olive oil, and season with ½ teaspoon of salt and black pepper.

2. Turn the squash, cut-side down, on the pan and roast until soft, about 45 to 50 minutes. Let it cool, then scoop out the flesh and discard the tough outer skin. Set aside.

3. Meanwhile, in a large stockpot over medium heat, heat the remaining 1 tablespoon of olive oil. Add the shallot and the remaining 1 teaspoon of salt. Cook, stirring often, until the shallot is softened and starting to turn golden at the edges, about 3 to 4 minutes.

4. Add the garlic and cook, stirring frequently, until fragrant, about 1 minute. Let the shallot-garlic mixture cool.

5. Transfer the squash and shallot-garlic mixture to a high-speed blender. Add the broth, maple syrup, vanilla (if using), and nutmeg. Blend until the mixture is smooth. (If you have a small blender, do this step in two batches.)

6. Transfer the soup to the stockpot over medium heat. Cook, stirring occasionally, until heated through. Divide the soup into bowls, drizzle each portion with ghee, and serve.

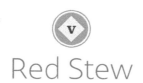

Red Stew

GLUTEN-FREE / VEGAN

PREP TIME: 15 MINUTES | COOK TIME: 35 MINUTES | SERVES 4

This stew is an Ayurvedic play on the big crowd pleaser called chili. The sweet potatoes sweeten and cool down the stronger flavors of the garlic and chili powder, and the adzuki beans add a good dose of vegan protein.

2 tablespoons extra-virgin olive oil

1 small onion, diced

2 garlic cloves, minced

2 small sweet potatoes, peeled and cubed

2 medium carrots, peeled and sliced

½ red bell pepper, chopped

1 (15-ounce) can adzuki beans, drained and rinsed

1 (15-ounce) can diced tomatoes with their juices or tomato sauce

½ cup vegetable broth

1 tablespoon chili powder

1 teaspoon ground cumin

½ teaspoon garlic powder or 1 large garlic clove, minced

½ teaspoon sea salt

¼ teaspoon freshly ground black pepper

1. In a stockpot over medium-high heat, heat the olive oil. Add the onion and garlic, and sauté for 1 to 2 minutes.

2. Add the sweet potatoes, carrots, and bell pepper, and continue to cook until the onion is soft, about 5 to 6 minutes.

3. Lower the heat to medium-low, and add the beans, tomatoes, broth, chili powder, cumin, garlic powder, salt, and black pepper. Stir to combine well.

4. Simmer, partially covered and stirring occasionally, for 20 to 25 minutes, until the flavors have mingled and the vegetables are cooked through.

5. Divide the soup into bowls and serve.

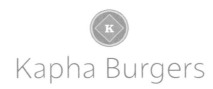

Kapha Burgers

GLUTEN-FREE / VEGAN

PREP TIME: 10 MINUTES | COOK TIME: 35 MINUTES | MAKES 2 BURGERS

This recipe is based on a traditional Indian recipe for veggie samosas, a yummy snack eaten on-the-go or as an appetizer in India. You'll want to sit down and savor this dish, though—you can even level up if you top it with a tiny bit of Indian mango pickle (see resources on page 158). It is spicy and sour and great for sluggish digestion. A little goes a long way, though, so just a tiny spoonful will do!

---

1 medium russet potato, peeled and chopped

1 tablespoon sunflower or corn oil, divided

1 teaspoon cumin seeds

¼ teaspoon coriander seeds

¾ teaspoon fennel seeds

1 to 1½ cups diced bell pepper, peas, corn, carrots, and finely chopped cauliflower

2 teaspoons grated peeled fresh ginger

½ teaspoon garam masala

½ teaspoon ground turmeric

½ teaspoon red chile powder or ground cayenne

½ teaspoon freshly squeezed lemon juice

Sea salt

¼ cup water

1 tablespoon cornmeal, plus more as needed

Indian mango pickle, for topping (optional)

1. In a small pot over medium-high heat, place the potato with enough water to cover it and bring to a boil. Cook for 10 minutes, until tender. Drain and set aside.

2. In a large skillet over medium heat, add ½ tablespoon of sunflower oil, and the cumin, coriander, and fennel. Cook, stirring occasionally, until the spices begin to brown, then add the vegetables and ginger. Sauté for 3 minutes, until the vegetables start to brown.

3. Add the garam masala, turmeric, chile powder, and lemon juice. Season to taste with salt, and stir to combine.

4. Add the water as needed to keep the mixture moist and slightly sticky, and continue to cook until the vegetables are fully tender, about 3 minutes. Remove from the heat.

5. Allow the vegetable mixture to cool slightly, then add the cooked potato. Mash in the potato until a dough-like consistency is formed. Transfer the mixture to a large bowl.

6. Add the cornmeal, and combine well until the mixture firms up and you are able to form patties.

7. In the same large skillet over medium heat, add the remaining ½ tablespoon of sunflower oil. Cook the patties on one side for 5 minutes, then flip them and cook the other side for 5 minutes, until each side is brown. Add extra oil as necessary to prevent them from sticking to the pan.

8. Top each burger with mango pickle (if using) and serve.

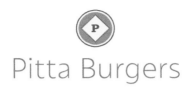

Pitta Burgers

GLUTEN-FREE / VEGAN

**PREP TIME: 15 MINUTES | COOK TIME: 30 MINUTES,
PLUS 15 TO 25 MINUTES TO CHILL | MAKES 4 BURGERS**

This is a great hearty lunch or dinner for Pitta people. My advice: Start cooking before you get hungry, so by the time you get hungry, your meal is ready to go. In fact, that should be a Pitta rule with all cooking.

¾ cup water

½ cup dry red lentils, rinsed well and drained

½ cup chopped tomato

⅓ teaspoon sea salt, plus more if needed

1 cup chopped broccoli (about ½-inch pieces)

1 (15-ounce) can pinto beans, drained and rinsed

½ teaspoon dried or 1 tablespoon minced fresh cilantro (optional)

½ teaspoon ground coriander

¼ teaspoon ground cumin

¼ cup finely chopped sweet onion

Few drops freshly squeezed lemon juice

3 to 4 tablespoons gluten-free bread crumbs

2 teaspoons coconut oil

Sliced avocado, for topping (optional)

1. In a medium saucepan over medium-low heat, combine the water, lentils, tomato, and salt, and bring to a simmer. Cook, stirring occasionally, for 10 minutes.

2. Add the broccoli, and stir to combine. Cook, stirring occasionally, for 10 to 12 minutes, or until the lentils are tender and all the liquid is gone. Remove from the heat, and cool slightly. Drain if there is excess water.

3. In a large bowl, combine the lentil mixture, beans, cilantro (if using), coriander, and cumin. Mix well so that most of the beans are well mashed. Add the onion and lemon juice, and mix well. Taste, and add additional salt as needed. The mixture will be soft. Chill in the freezer for 15 minutes or in the refrigerator for 25 minutes.

4. Add the bread crumbs, and combine well until the mixture firms up and you are able to form patties.

5. In a medium skillet over medium heat, heat the coconut oil. Cook the patties on one side for 3 to 4 minutes, then flip and cook the other side for 3 to 4 minutes, until each side is brown. (You can also bake them in a 400°F oven for 20 minutes, then flip and bake for an additional 5 to 10 minutes.)

6. Top each burger with sliced avocado (if using), and serve.

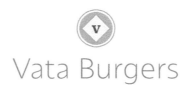

Vata Burgers

GLUTEN-FREE / VEGAN

PREP TIME: 45 MINUTES | COOK TIME: 25 MINUTES | MAKES 4 TO 6 BURGERS

Quinoa is a staple in my kitchen. It's full of protein and slow-burning carbohydrates for stamina. My father loves it as well, although he calls it "qween-wah," which is always entertaining. My nickname for this one is the "Eat a Sweet Potato and Get Back to Me Burger," because sweet potatoes are grounding medicine if you're feeling spaced out.

Coconut oil or ghee, for greasing

¾ cup quinoa

¾ cup dried red lentils, cooked according to package instructions

2 roasted sweet potatoes, mashed

1 teaspoon ground cumin

1 teaspoon paprika

½ teaspoon chili powder

Sea salt

Freshly ground black pepper

Cilantro Chutney, for topping (optional, page 85)

1. Preheat the oven to 375°F. Grease a baking sheet with coconut oil.

2. In a large bowl, combine the quinoa, lentils, sweet potatoes, cumin, paprika, and chili powder. Season to taste with salt and black pepper. Mix well.

3. Form the mixture into 4 to 6 patties. Transfer the patties to the prepared baking sheet, and bake for 12 minutes. Flip the patties, and bake on the other side for another 12 minutes.

4. Top each burger with chutney (if using), and serve.

Chachi Luna's Green Tara Sauce

GLUTEN-FREE / VEGAN
PREP TIME: 5 MINUTES | MAKES 1 CUP

Chachi was a student of mine. She loved to cook. She called nutritional yeast "hippie flakes" and used them in a lot of her recipes. This one is my favorite. It's so tasty, you could eat it on its own or over anything—it would make cardboard taste yummy! Best for Kapha and Pitta types, its rawness could be tough for Vata.

1 large handful fresh cilantro leaves

1 large handful baby arugula

¼ cup raw pumpkin seeds

¼ cup raw sunflower seeds

1 tablespoon nutritional yeast

1 tablespoon apple cider vinegar or freshly squeezed lemon juice, plus more as needed

Dash hot sauce (Kapha only)

Sea salt

1. In a high-speed blender or food processor, combine the cilantro, baby arugula, pumpkin seeds, sunflower seeds, nutritional yeast, vinegar, and hot sauce. Season to taste with salt. Purée, adding water, until the mixture is smooth and creamy.

2. Taste, and add additional salt and vinegar as needed.

3. Transfer the sauce to a jar with a lid, and store in the refrigerator for up to two days.

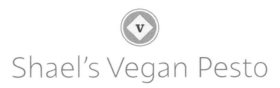

Shael's Vegan Pesto

GLUTEN-FREE / VEGAN
PREP TIME: 5 MINUTES | MAKES 1½ CUPS

My dear friend Shael Berni is one of the most loving, generous people I know. She went to culinary school and is always taking traditional recipes and making them vegan and healthy. Here's her contribution. The umeboshi plum paste (see resources, page 158) is a Japanese ingredient, and a little goes a long way. According to Ayurveda, it is primarily the sour taste, which is best for Vata types, but a little bit is fine for Kapha and Pitta. Try serving this pesto over pasta, cooked veggies, grains, or veggie burgers, or as a dip for crackers or vegetables.

2½ cups packed fresh basil leaves

¾ cup extra-virgin olive oil

¼ cup toasted walnuts

3 garlic cloves, peeled

1½ teaspoons umeboshi pickled plum paste

1. In a high-speed blender or food processor, combine the basil, oil, walnuts, garlic, and plum paste, blending until smooth.

2. Transfer the pesto to a jar with a lid, and store in the refrigerator for up to three days.

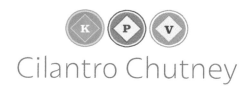

Cilantro Chutney

GLUTEN-FREE / VEGAN

PREP TIME: 5 MINUTES | MAKES 1½ CUPS

David Shemesh and his wife, Elian, are the founders of WOOM Center, one of the two studios I teach at in New York City. David was a chef and owned successful restaurants before he "went yoga" and opened Woom. This chutney is full of bright flavor and color. It's good for all doshas, but Vata types should reduce the garlic to one small clove. This tastes great over pasta, veggies, grains, and veggie burgers, or as a dip for crackers or vegetables.

1 cup extra-virgin olive oil

1 large handful fresh cilantro leaves, rinsed well in cold water

1 small handful fresh mint leaves, rinsed well in cold water

1 small handful fresh Italian parsley, rinsed well in cold water

2 small garlic cloves, peeled

Juice of ½ lemon

Sea salt

Freshly ground black pepper

1. In a high-speed blender or food processor, combine the olive oil, cilantro, mint, parsley, garlic, and lemon juice. Season to taste with salt and black pepper. Purée until the mixture is smooth.

2. Transfer the chutney to a jar with a lid, and store in the refrigerator for up to two days.

Kapha Spicy Seed Snack

GLUTEN-FREE / VEGAN

PREP TIME: 5 MINUTES | COOK TIME: 15 MINUTES | MAKES 1 CUP

Back in 2014, I was hired to co-lead the first yoga teacher training program in Khartoum, Sudan. My dear friend Nada, who lives in Khartoum, is Ethiopian, and she and her mother gave me an Ethiopian cooking lesson. It was then that I fell in love with berbere, a traditional Ethiopian spice blend containing anywhere from 10 to 15 different spices. It's pungent without being burn-your-mouth-off hot—great for Kapha dosha. I've seen it recently at a local grocery store, or you can find it online (see resources on page 158). It's worth tracking down, I promise you.

½ cup raw sunflower seeds

½ cup raw pumpkin seeds

2 teaspoons sunflower oil

1 teaspoon berbere

1. Preheat the oven to 350°F.

2. In a medium bowl, combine the sunflower seeds and pumpkin seeds. Add the sunflower oil and berbere, tossing to coat.

3. Transfer the seed mixture to a baking sheet, and spread evenly. Roast for 12 to 15 minutes, stirring once.

4. Transfer the seed snack to a jar with a lid, and store at room temperature for up to three days.

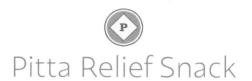

Pitta Relief Snack

GLUTEN-FREE / VEGAN
PREP TIME: 5 MINUTES | COOK TIME: 20 MINUTES | SERVES 2

My teacher Dana Flynn makes these all the time. They are perfect as a sweet treat to nibble on when dinner is a few hours away. Take a break and have a few with a cup of mint or chamomile tea.

1 large sweet potato, washed well and cut into ½-inch disks

1 to 2 teaspoons melted coconut oil

1 teaspoon Pitta Masala (page 65) or ½ teaspoon ground cinnamon

1. Preheat the oven to 350°F.

2. Place the sweet potato on a baking sheet, and drizzle with the coconut oil, tossing to coat. Arrange the slices on the baking sheet so there is space between each of them. Sprinkle with the masala.

3. Bake for 5 to 10 minutes. Flip the slices, and bake on the other side for 5 to 10 minutes more, until soft in the center.

4. Serve and enjoy right away.

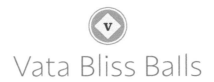

Vata Bliss Balls

GLUTEN-FREE / VEGAN
PREP TIME: 15 MINUTES | MAKES 15 TO 20 BALLS

These are sweet and rich with protein, healthy fats, and fiber for irregular Vata digestion. Make sure you get cashews that taste fresh—nuts that hang around grocery stores too long can spoil.

2 cups raw cashews

1 cup Medjool dates

¼ cup cacao powder

2 tablespoons hemp seeds

2 tablespoons cacao nibs

Dash apple cider vinegar

1 tablespoon goji berries (optional)

1 tablespoon coconut flakes (optional)

1 tablespoon vegan protein powder (optional)

Coconut flour or cacao powder, for rolling (optional)

1. In a high-speed blender or food processor, combine the cashews, dates, cacao, hemp seeds, cacao nibs, and vinegar. Add the goji berries (if using), coconut flakes (if using), and protein powder (if using). Blend until the mixture forms a paste.

2. Remove the mixture from the blender, and roll into 2-inch balls. Roll each ball in coconut flour (if using).

3. Store in the refrigerator in an airtight container for up to three days.

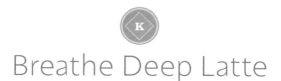

Breathe Deep Latte

GLUTEN-FREE / VEGETARIAN
PREP TIME: 5 MINUTES | COOK TIME: 5 MINUTES | SERVES 1

This beverage is helpful as an expectorant—to get mucus out of the lungs. It's perfect for that damp, cold, late-winter Kapha evening.

1 cup organic dairy or almond milk

1 dried bay leaf

¾ teaspoon freshly ground black pepper

¾ teaspoon ground ginger

¾ teaspoon ground cardamom

3-finger pinch ground cinnamon

3-finger pinch ground star anise

1 teaspoon honey

1. In a small saucepan over medium-low heat, combine the milk, bay leaf, black pepper, ginger, cardamom, cinnamon, and star anise, and bring to a gentle simmer. Cook for 5 minutes.

2. Remove from the heat, and add the honey right before drinking.

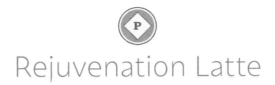

Rejuvenation Latte

GLUTEN-FREE / VEGAN
PREP TIME: 5 MINUTES | SERVES 1

My Pitta latte has dates for sweetness and uses almond milk. You could also make this really decadent by using half almond milk and half coconut milk.

1 cup almond milk

2 Medjool dates

1 (1-inch) piece fresh ginger, peeled, or pinch saffron

5-finger pinch ground cinnamon

1. In a high-speed blender, combine the milk, dates, ginger, and cinnamon, and blend until frothy.

2. Enjoy at room temperature.

Calm Down Latte
(Golden Milk)

GLUTEN-FREE / VEGETARIAN

PREP TIME: 5 MINUTES | COOK TIME: 5 MINUTES | SERVES 1 GENEROUSLY

Best for Vata types, this latte may be used by other doshas for calming excess Vata. Golden Milk has gotten a lot of play in recent years, and I'm glad to hear it! Turmeric has been shown to be helpful for the nervous system, and it's antibacterial, digestive, and anti-inflammatory. Ashwagandha (see resources, page 158) is an Ayurvedic herb that's an adaptogen. Adaptogens help the body function well in times of stress. Here's my recipe; feel free to embellish. I like to use a mix of almond and coconut milk. It's very soothing anytime, but especially nice before bed.

1½ cups organic dairy or nondairy milk

¼ teaspoon ground turmeric

⅛ teaspoon ground cinnamon

5-finger pinch powdered ashwagandha root

3-finger pinch freshly ground black pepper

3-finger pinch ground ginger

3-finger pinch freshly ground nutmeg

Dash maple syrup or 3-finger pinch coconut sugar (if using dairy milk)

1. In a small saucepan over low heat, combine the milk, turmeric, cinnamon, ashwagandha, black pepper, ginger, and nutmeg. Cook, stirring occasionally, until heated through.

2. Remove from the heat, and add the maple syrup (if using dairy milk) right before drinking. Nondairy milks tend to be sweet enough without it.

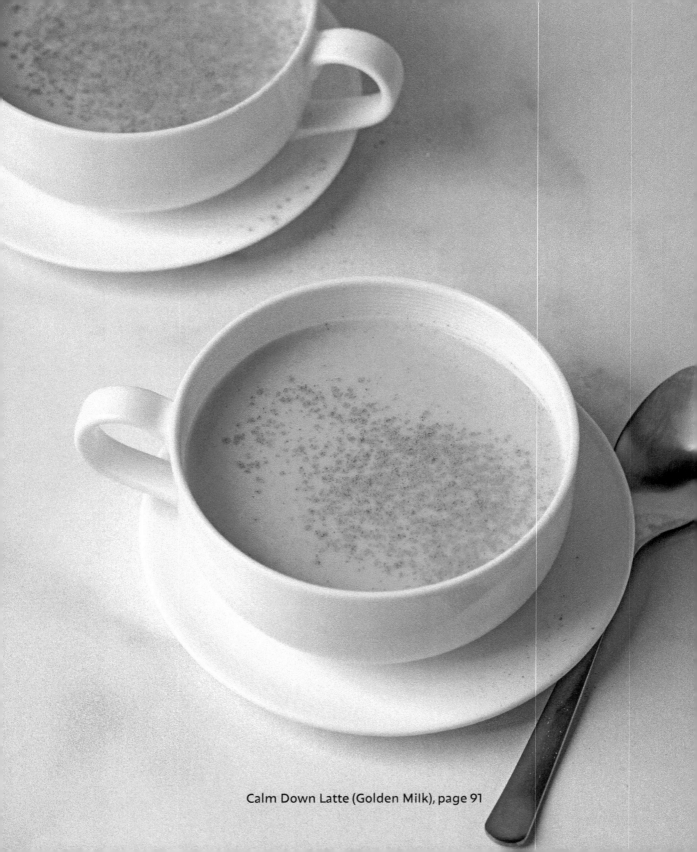

Calm Down Latte (Golden Milk), page 91

Seasonal Ayurvedic Menus

Here are some menus for the seasons. You can easily double the lunch or dinner recipes and invite some friends to join you!

Kapha Day	Pitta Day	Vata Day
Breakfast: Chickpea pancakes (see page 62)	**Breakfast:** Pitta smoothie with fresh blueberries (see page 63), mint tea	**Breakfast:** Bring-Me-Back Kichadi (see page 60), tulsi tea
Snack: Spicy chai black tea	**Lunch:** Cool-It-Down Kichadi (see page 59)	**Lunch:** Orange Soup (see page 72) and stir-fried baby greens with sesame oil and soy sauce
Lunch: Grain bowl with millet, Veggie Stir-Fry (see page 70), and Chachi Luna's Green Tara Sauce (see page 83)	**Snack:** Rejuvenation Latte (see page 90)	**Snack:** Vata Bliss Balls (see page 88)
Snack: Kapha Spicy Seed Snack (see page 86) or popcorn with a pinch of berbere or masala	**Dinner:** Pitta Burger (see page 80)	**Dinner:** More kichadi or pasta (gluten-free if desired) with Shael's Vegan Pesto (see page 84)
Dinner: Kapha Burger (see page 78) with Cilantro Chutney (see page 85)	**Dessert:** Fresh coconut pieces	**Before Bed:** Calm Down Latte (see page 91)

Food Guidelines by Dosha

Here's a simple, at-a-glance list to help you determine which foods are best for each dosha. Keep in mind that if one dosha is presenting strongly on you, it's best to follow those food rules no matter the season. Otherwise, follow the guidelines of the season with an eye toward your own dosha. For example:

- Feeling very Vata going into Kapha season, stick with Vata foods.
- Feeling pretty balanced going into Kapha season, eat more from the Kapha foods list, and if you start to feel out of balance, adjust to your own dosha.

	Kapha dosha, and useful for all in Kapha season	Pitta dosha, and useful for all in Pitta season	Vata dosha, and useful for all in Vata season
FRUIT	apples, berries, cherries, cranberries, figs, lemons, limes, peaches, pears, pomegranates, prunes, raisins	apples (sweet), apricots, avocado, berries, cherries, coconut, dates, figs, grapes, lime, mangoes, melons, oranges (sweet), papaya, pears, pineapple (sweet), plums, pomegranates, prunes, raisins, watermelons	*Dried fruit may be eaten if soaked first.* apples (cooked), apricots, avocado, bananas, berries, cherries, dates (fresh), figs (fresh), grapefruit, grapes, kiwi, lemons, limes, mangoes, melons, oranges, papaya, peaches, pineapple, plums

	Kapha dosha, and useful for all in Kapha season	Pitta dosha, and useful for all in Pitta season	Vata dosha, and useful for all in Vata season
VEGETABLES	artichoke, asparagus, beets, broccoli, Brussels sprouts, burdock, cabbage, carrots, cauliflower, celery, corn, daikon radish, dandelion greens, eggplant, fennel, garlic, green beans, green chile peppers, kale, leafy greens, leeks, mushrooms, okra, onions, peas, peppers, radishes, spinach, sprouts, summer squash, tomatoes (cooked), turnips, white potatoes	artichoke, asparagus, beets (cooked), broccoli, Brussels sprouts, cabbage, carrots, cauliflower, celery, cucumber, dandelion greens, fennel, green beans, kale, leafy greens, lettuce, mushrooms, okra, olives (black), onions (cooked for extra sweetness only), parsnips, peas, sweet peppers, potatoes (sweet and white), pumpkin, radishes (cooked), squashes, zucchini	*Best to cook vegetables in general. Sweet soft lettuce may be eaten raw.* asparagus, beets, carrots, cauliflower (occasional), cucumber (raw, cut out seeds), fennel, garlic (cooked only), green beans, leafy greens (occasional), leeks, lettuce (occasional), okra, olives (black), onions (cooked only), parsnip, peas, potatoes (sweet), pumpkin, radishes (cooked), spinach (cooked and raw, occasional), squash (summer and winter), zucchini
GRAINS	amaranth, barley, buckwheat, cereal (dry, puffed), corn, crackers, millet, muesli, oats, polenta, quinoa, rice (basmati, wild), rye	amaranth, barley, cereal (preferably oat based), couscous, crackers, oats (cooked), rice (basmati, white, wild), wheat	amaranth (occasional), oats (cooked), quinoa, rice (all), wheat (if tolerated)

	Kapha dosha, and useful for all in Kapha season	Pitta dosha, and useful for all in Pitta season	Vata dosha, and useful for all in Vata season
LEGUMES	adzuki beans, black beans, chickpeas, lentils (red and brown), mung beans, navy beans, pinto beans, split peas, tofu (cooked well)	adzuki beans, black beans, chickpeas, kidney beans, lentils (red and brown), mung beans, navy beans, pinto beans, soybeans (edamame, tofu, tempeh), split peas, white beans	lentils (red, occasional), mung beans, peanuts (occasional), tofu (occasional)
NUTS AND SEEDS	*Nuts aren't recommended.* chia, flax, popcorn (no salt or oil/butter), pumpkin seeds, sunflower seeds	almonds, coconut, flax, popcorn (coconut oil or ghee, no salt), pumpkin seeds, sunflower seeds	almonds, brazil nuts, cashews, coconut, hazelnuts, macadamia nuts, pecans, pine nuts, pistachios, walnuts; chia, flax, pumpkin seeds; sesame seeds, sunflower seeds
OILS	almond, corn, ghee, sesame (external use), sunflower	avocado, coconut, ghee, olive, flaxseed	avocado, coconut, ghee, olive, sesame

	Kapha dosha, and useful for all in Kapha season	Pitta dosha, and useful for all in Pitta season	Vata dosha, and useful for all in Vata season
SPICES AND HERBS	*All are good. Go easy on the salt; it's not recommended for Kapha types.*	basil (fresh), cardamom (occasional), cilantro, cinnamon, coriander, cumin, dill, fennel, ginger (fresh), mint, parsley (occasional), peppermint, saffron, spearmint, turmeric	allspice, anise, asafoetida (hing), basil, bay leaves, black pepper, cardamom, cilantro, cinnamon, cloves, coriander, cumin, dill, fennel, ginger, mint, mustard seeds, nutmeg, oregano, paprika (sweet), parsley, rosemary, saffron, salt, tarragon, thyme, turmeric, vanilla
SWEETENER	honey (raw, organic)	coconut sugar, maple syrup, rice syrup	barley malt, coconut sugar, honey (raw, organic), molasses, rice syrup, turbinado
ANIMAL FOODS	buttermilk, ghee, goat cheese, sour yogurt (as opposed to Greek, thick), white chicken, eggs, freshwater fish, shrimp, white turkey	butter (unsalted), cheese (soft, fresh, unsalted), cottage cheese, cow's milk, ghee, goat's milk and cheese, ice cream, yogurt (occasional use, stay with the varieties like unsweetened Greek yogurt, which is much less sour than other varieties, or dilute the yogurt with water), chicken (white), egg (whites), fish (freshwater), turkey (white)	butter, buttermilk, cheese (hard occasional, soft whenever), cottage cheese, cow's milk, ghee, goat cheese, ice cream (occasional), sour cream (occasional), yogurt (add digestive spices), chicken (dark whenever, white occasional), eggs, fish (all kinds), seafood

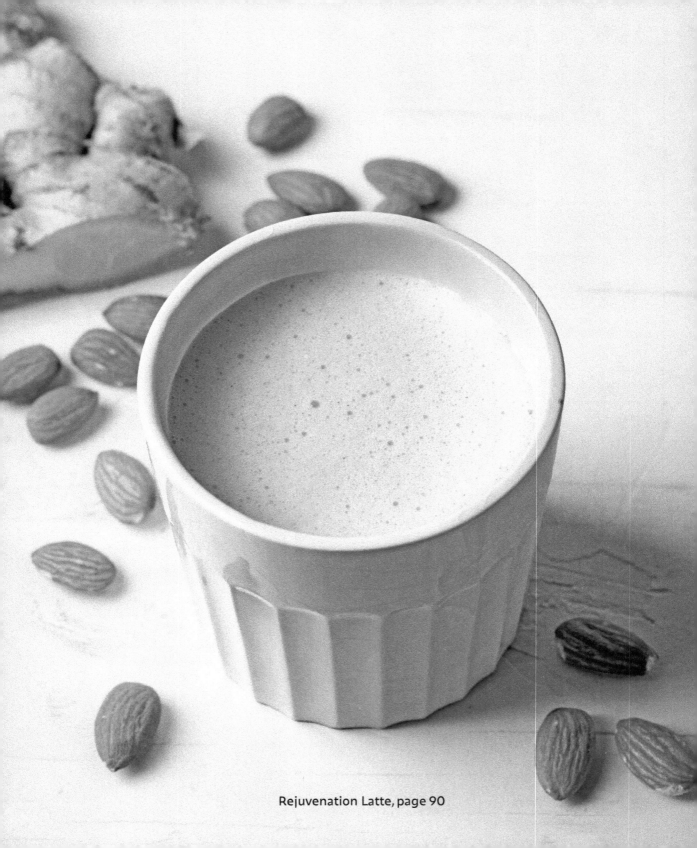

Rejuvenation Latte, page 90

5

REMEDIES AND PRACTICES FOR SPECIFIC AILMENTS

In this chapter, we will discuss simple Ayurvedic remedies for common ailments. As mentioned in chapter 1, these are not replacements for regularly seeing a medical practitioner, but my hope is that with the shifts we can make to our lifestyles, ailments can be alleviated. Partner the remedies specific to your needs with the other suggestions for your dosha, and implement a plan for optimal health and well-being. Remember that holistic health is not designed to work overnight: Trust the process, and you will see slow, steady shifts.

Digestive Problems

Digestive problems can be an issue for any dosha. Sometimes, a student will approach me and say, "Ali, I have digestive problems. What should I do?" My usual answer is "Book a consultation." Digestive problems are so ubiquitous and broad ranging, it's impossible to give a recommendation without diving deeper. Read on for specific symptoms, and see which category feels accurate to your needs.

Agni Accelerator

SYMPTOMS: Slow digestion and no appetite (Kapha and Vata)

TRY THIS: Have a small, ½-inch piece of fresh ginger with a squeeze of lemon juice and a sprinkle of sea salt 30 minutes before meals.

Aloe Me Tonic

SYMPTOMS: Acid reflux, acid indigestion (Pitta)

TRY THIS: Twice a day, drink a half cup of room-temperature water mixed with ¼ cup of pure aloe juice, ½ cup raw organic coconut water, and a handful of crushed mint leaves.

Tummy Soother Tea

SYMPTOMS: Gas, bloating, constipation (Vata)

TRY THIS: Brew up a strong cup of digestive tea: Combine 1 teaspoon of fennel seeds, 1 teaspoon of crushed mint leaves, and 1 teaspoon of minced fresh ginger in 2 cups of water. Simmer for 10 minutes, strain, and drink right after dinner.

Movement Medicine

My first suggestion is to find an exercise practice you enjoy. Movement should not be something that feels like punishment! There are so many different classes and online options, and you don't need to spend hours in a gym to see benefits. In fact, too much exercise can be taxing on the adrenals and mess up your system. Try to do more walking, and take the stairs instead of the elevator. A few times a week, do at least 30 minutes of something that gets your heart pumping a bit. (Kapha people, try to do it four or five times a week if possible.) This could be a gentle jog outside, a dance fitness class with a friend, an online yoga practice, a swim if you have access to a pool, or anything else you enjoy. Take your dog (or a friend's) for a romp, hike a nearby trail, or join a volleyball team. The possibilities are endless, so feel free to mix it up! See the kickstart plans on page 110 for more dosha-specific exercise recommendations.

Night Trip

To aid your liver with detoxification, take ½ teaspoon of triphala in warm water every night before bed.

Spice Me Up

If you find you have a sugar craving, load up on cinnamon. In addition to helping with cravings, cinnamon freshens breath, helps with digestion, and has been proven to help support cholesterol reduction. Make cinnamon tea by combining 2 broken cinnamon sticks in 2 cups of water and simmering for 10 minutes. Strain and drink. You can have up to 3 cups a day. You can also put a few drops of cinnamon essential oil in a diffuser.

Anxiety

Anxiety is usually a Vata condition. Today, anxiety can strike any of us as family and/or work pressures mount.

Music Medicine

Keep music soothing and gentle. Try some soft classical music or rhythmic percussion. My favorites are Morley, Masood Ali Khan, and Zoë Keating for those times when I feel tense.

Go for Gold

Make Golden Milk (see page 91) and enjoy in a quiet corner.

Holy Pause

Take a restorative yoga class, or look online for a restorative sequence and do it at home. Even five minutes in constructive rest is helpful. Get a pillow for under your head, and lie on your back with your knees bent and feet on the ground. Place your feet slightly wider than your outer hips, and bring your knees together to touch. Let your hands rest on the lowest part of your belly with your elbows draped over your sides. Close your eyes, and breathe deeply. If closing your eyes makes you more anxious, leave them open.

Smells Like Peace

Essential oils have been a game changer for me. I have a diffuser in my bedroom, another one in my living room, and I carry them with me all day long. Some oils that are good for anxiety are lavender, chamomile, clary sage, sandalwood, rose, neroli, and cedarwood—the list goes on and on!

Depression

Depression is usually a Kapha condition. Sometimes, it's possible to go so far into Vata or Pitta imbalance that you crash and mild depression can creep in. All the more reason to try to stay in balance when you can. Here are some things that can lessen or shorten this dis-ease.

Citrus Sparkler

In your essential oil diffuser, add 2 drops each of lemon, wild orange, and bergamot essential oils. Don't have a diffuser? Get a clean glass jar and put the same recipe in a cup of carrier oil such as jojoba or fractionated coconut oil. Use for your abhyanga massage or dab some on your wrists, temples, and bottoms of your feet.

Sunshine of My Life

Get some sunshine—it stimulates the production of melatonin in the pineal gland, which helps support both immunity and mood. Get outside in fresh air. If it's really cold, bundle up well, but don't avoid getting out of your house.

Beginner's Mind

Try something you've never done, or something you haven't done in years. Take a Hula-Hoop class, go ice-skating with a friend, or call a few friends and go bowling or hiking. We can get stuck in a rut so easily, and each day can seem like all the others. If you can take a personal day, do it. Go to a museum, take yourself out for lunch, get your nails done, or get a massage. Staycations can be extraordinary for a reset!

Insomnia

Kapha people usually sleep soundly. Insomnia is generally a Pitta or Vata imbalance. Sleep is vital for the body to repair itself and for the mind to reset. Try these suggestions to improve the quality and quantity of your slumber.

Early to Bed

If at all possible, try to be in bed as close to Kapha time of day as possible, around 10:00 p.m. If that's not possible, at least try to make it to bed before midnight. If you aren't used to going to bed early, try it for just one night. Get in bed at 9:30 p.m., and read a little or do a yoga nidra. Yoga nidra is a type of guided relaxation, done in Savasana, which is a comfortable pose lying on your back. You can find many versions of it online; find one that is appealing to you. It's a lovely way to drift off. Have the sound loud enough to just barely hear it, and have lights out by 10:00 p.m.

Power Down

Turn off all electronics at least an hour before bedtime. That includes your TV, computer, tablet, and phone. Move the phone away from your nightstand, and replace it with a clock. Establish a discipline around it.

Digestion Reset

Try not to eat at least two hours before bed, don't have more than one alcoholic beverage, and resist the urge to drink caffeine past noon. All of these factors can contribute to unsettled sleep.

Go for Gold

Have a cup of Golden Milk (see page 91) before bed, and add a little extra nutmeg to it. Nutmeg is a natural soporific.

Eczema

Oh, eczema folks. There is a special place in my heart for you. I was the kid covered in rashes on a regular basis. They were in the crooks of my inner arms, the backs of my knees, sometimes on my neck. They were so itchy and embarrassing to me as a child! My parents knew nothing about Ayurveda, and I ate tons of peanut butter sandwiches (inflammatory) and drank gallons of grapefruit juice (too much of the sour taste). Plus, I was in tight polyester dance clothes all the time! Ayurveda has helped me tremendously with this. Eczema is an autoimmune disease, which puts it in Pitta territory, but Vata is there, too, as it helps to fan the flames. Here's what works for me.

More Coconut, More Better
Focus on your diet, first and foremost. Follow a Pitta-pacifying diet (see the lists on page 94).

Aloe Me
Twice a day, drink ½ cup of room-temperature water mixed with ¼ cup of pure aloe juice, ½ cup of raw organic coconut water, and a handful of crushed mint leaves.

Go Bare
Remove all jewelry, especially necklaces if your neck is showing signs of eczema.

Skin Solution
Wear only natural fibers next to your skin: cotton, linen, cashmere, or silk. Anything else can be aggravating. If it's really bad, make a soothing paste by putting a big handful of cilantro leaves in a blender with ½ cup of water and blending thoroughly, then apply to clean skin. Leave the paste on for 15 minutes, then gently rinse.

Dry, Cracked Skin

Dry, cracked sin is usually a Vata condition from extreme temperatures—whether cold or hot. Here are two different methods for healing. I recommend you do both.

It's an Inside Job

Skin issues should always be initially treated from the inside. Follow a Vata-soothing diet (see the lists on page 94). Add foods with good fats like avocados, almond or coconut butter, and extra-virgin olive oil. Eat some full-fat plain yogurt or cottage cheese if you tolerate dairy well. If not, try a coconut-, cashew-, or almond-based yogurt, and add some hemp seeds for omega-3 oils. Get some shatavari (see resources on page 158). It is an Ayurvedic herb from the asparagus family that has been shown to support the body's function in stressful times. It is especially helpful with imbalanced Vata conditions, as it also supports a woman's menstrual cycle (especially for Vata) at all phases of her life, including easing menopause symptoms. Take as directed.

It's an Outside Job

Make a sugar scrub with 1 cup of natural sugar, ½ cup of sesame oil, and a couple drops of lavender essential oil. Do a gentle scrub on affected areas to get off any old, scaly skin. Follow with abhyanga massage with sesame oil. Try not to take superhot showers. Water should be kept at a warm temperature. Make sure your bodywash or soap is super gentle, natural, and creamy. And don't overdo it; soap can strip away your skin's natural protective coating.

Hair Care

Kapha people often have the advantage here—their inherent heartiness can be a source of beautiful, thick, shiny hair. For the rest of us, there are ways to take care of what we do have to keep our hair and scalp in good condition.

Mane Event

I don't know about you, but my hair changes on the regular. I have dyed it black, bleached it platinum, straightened it with straightening irons, curled it with curling irons, braided it, blew it out—the works! No wonder it can get limp and lifeless. That sexy JLo blowout you've been sporting or the fauxhawk with all the gel and spray can wreak havoc on your hair. These days, I know simple is better. I almost never use a blow-dryer anymore. That being said, I teach yoga most days, so a basic ponytail is better for me than anything that requires a lot of upkeep. Once a month or so, I coat my hair in coconut oil, starting with the ends and working my way up. Try it, and while you're at it, give yourself a good scalp massage—it's very stimulating for hair follicles. If you've ever been on the receiving end of a good scalp massage, you know how heavenly it can be. Give that to yourself—it's so loving!

Flake No More

For dandruff, add 1 tablespoon of neem oil and 2 drops each of rosemary, peppermint, and lavender essential oils to some coconut oil and leave the oil on your scalp for a few hours or overnight, if possible. If you're doing that, definitely put an old towel or T-shirt over your pillowcase. If your hair is long, pile it in a loose ponytail on top of your head. You will sleep like a baby that night. In the morning, rinse it a couple of times and then shampoo.

Facial Care

The skin on your face is delicate. Harsh soaps and too much scrubbing can strip it bare and make dry skin irritated. Harsh soaps can also irritate acne. Here are some recommendations based on dosha. If you resonate more with a dosha that differs from your own, feel free to follow that skin care regimen instead. Sometimes, percentages of dosha can present in different ways (e.g., if you're Vata-Pitta but your skin is more Pitta than Vata). Each dosha can benefit from facial massage—here are directions.

Facial Massage How-To

1. Using the tips of your fingers, apply your dosha oil and make gentle circles around your eye sockets.
2. Rub the oil into your forehead, stroking up and out toward your hairline above your ears.
3. Skip your nose unless you've been in the sun.

4. Make some circles with the flat of your palm on your cheeks.
5. Make circles around your mouth with your fingertips.
6. Apply the dosha oil to your neck, again stroking upward, this time with your full hand.
7. Rub any excess oil into your hands, especially around your nail beds.

Kapha Skin

CONDITION: Oily, congested skin

TRY THIS: Every day, cleanse gently with a warm washcloth, and add a drop of tea tree oil to your facial cleanser, which should be one that is specifically designed for oily skin. Your facial oil should be jojoba with 1 drop each of bergamot, clary sage, and lavender. You can also do the facial massage described previously. A bentonite clay mask once a week is great for you. Put a tablespoon of clay powder in a metal or glass bowl. Add 1 teaspoon each of neem powder (see resources, page 158) and raw organic honey, and stir well. Add enough water to make a paste, and spread in a thin layer over your face. Leave to dry for 5 minutes or so, and then remove with a warm washcloth.

Pitta Skin

CONDITION: Red, inflamed, sensitive skin

TRY THIS: Be careful, Pitta people! Your skin might get hives or rashes from food or fabric sensitivity—I even once had a reaction to hair products from a trip to the salon. Here's what to do, and it's a nice practice for once a week as well. Wet a soft, cotton washcloth, and place it in the freezer for a few minutes. Take it out and hold it over your face, especially your eyes. (Your eyes can get very inflamed with all the technology you use on a daily basis, so cooling them off should feel refreshing.) Once a month, do a clay mask. Combine 2 tablespoons of bentonite clay with 1 teaspoon each of sandalwood powder and neem powder (see resources, page 158). Add enough water or milk to make a paste, then apply it to your face in a very thin coat. Leave the mask on for 5 minutes or so, then remove it with a soft, cool washcloth. After, put some face oil on and massage it in, following the facial massage described on page 106. You can use a base oil of almond with a couple drops of vitamin E. If you have blemishes, add 2 drops each of lavender oil and tea tree oil. If you are blemish free, add 2 drops each of lavender oil and sandalwood oil. You can benefit from a spritz of rose water as well—it smells wonderful and is cooling and nourishing for your skin. Make sure you get a brand that is free of chemicals and preservatives.

Vata Skin

CONDITION: Dry, lifeless-looking skin

TRY THIS: Vata skin usually needs a lot of moisture and gentle cleansing. Use a soft washcloth with warm water and a creamy cleanser in the morning and evening. After cleansing, pour 4 or 5 drops each of rose hip seed oil and vitamin E oil in to your palm, and add 2 drops each of geranium oil and rose oil. Then follow the facial massage described on page 106.

Body Care

Abhyanga is a loving and beautiful act of self-care.

All-Over Body Massage

Oil yourself up on a daily basis so your skin stays nourished and healthy. Start at your feet and work your way up, with extra circles around the joints and a firm massage around your belly in a clockwise direction. Pick a couple of essential oils you like, and start with 1 or 2 drops in your base oil—the best one for Vata types is sesame. Remember, you can always add more essential oil, but if you put in too much to start off with, it can aggravate the skin.

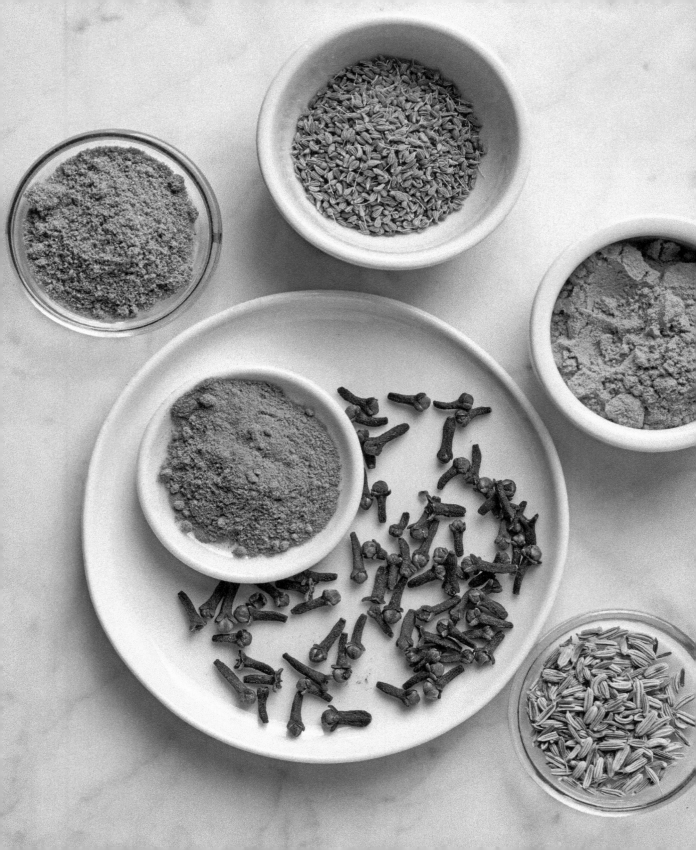

PART TWO

KICKSTART PLANS

WE HAVE GONE THROUGH A LITTLE HISTORY, broken down the major theories, and covered some of the most common issues related to Ayurvedic balance. Now it's time to take action. The following chapters provide clear, one-week plans to help you start integrating these ancient theories into your twenty-first century life. On the following pages you will find a weeklong kickstart plan for each dosha, with food and exercise suggestions, journaling, and more. Consider this your invitation to commit to one week of prioritizing your self-care and diving in to living modern Ayurveda. I recommend that you read through the week carefully before you start and that you be honest with yourself about whether the time is right for you to dive in. You should not be traveling, hosting houseguests, or facing an intense workweek during your kickstart. Give yourself the time and space to be able to follow through on your commitment.

Ayurvedic Rules to Live By

I took a weeklong training with Judith Lasater, who is responsible for the restorative yoga movement in the United States. She is one of the founders of *Yoga Journal*, has written incredible books, and has been teaching since 1971. One of the greatest moments of the training was her four recommendations for lasting health and well-being.

+ **No rushing.** In my mind, that means manage your time well. I find that, if I am rushing, 99.9 percent of the time it's because I have been unrealistic about my time management. Sometimes life throws us an unexpected challenge, like a horrific traffic jam or stalled subway. But sometimes, we just got stuck on a call that we should've figured out how to exit gracefully, or we spent too much time scrolling Instagram or lingering at work or the gym just because we were spacing out—not because we were working or working out productively. What I try to do now is notice when I am rushing and figure out where I miscalculated. Rushing sucks. You feel anxious, your adrenals go on alert, and if you are late, the barrage of lame excuses never feels good. None of this is good for staying peaceful and calm.

+ **No waiting.** You can wait, but you don't get to wait. Meaning, no checking the time obsessively, sighing loudly, or complaining about the "damn elevator/train/tourists/405 South!" In India, there is a myth about the god Shiva, who was always accompanied by his faithful companion, the bull Nandi. When you go to Shiva temples, there are statues of Nandi sitting outside. Nandi represents honor, faith, and wisdom. One of my teachers said we should see Nandi seated outside the temple as a reminder that patience is a virtue, that we can wait quietly and respectfully. And really, doesn't this align with the first rule? Often impatience comes from mismanaging time and feeling like we are going to be late, which leads to rushing. Once I was in India, and I wanted to buy some food for children begging in Rishikesh. The restaurant I ran into to get them a meal was taking *forever*. I was concerned the children would leave the area, so I was anxious and impatient as I stood outside the restaurant—probably rolling my eyes at the cashier. Then, I tuned in enough to the moment to realize that the Gayatri mantra, a very beautiful and holy mantra, was playing loudly enough from the store next door for me to hear it. I literally felt my mind shift with the thought, "Well, I could wait and be completely restless, impatient, and rude, or I could wait and chant along with the mantra and enjoy the sunshine on my face." I was lucky something came along to bring me back to sanity. We don't always get so lucky, so it's up to us to develop the necessary skills to bring peace without divine intervention (although that skill *is* divine intervention, if you ask me). So, no rushing, and no waiting.

♦ **Pause daily.** Do one restorative yoga pose every day for at least 10 minutes. Full transparency: I don't do it every day. I try to do it a few times a week, especially on those days when I don't do yoga. Those times when I skip it, it's more about trying to figure out why I "don't have the time," or don't prioritize my own well-being enough. You don't need fancy yoga equipment. Even if you are in the middle of a busy day, you know you would be more productive and clearer if you found a quiet corner somewhere at some point and lay down and put your legs up the wall. Even five minutes makes a difference.

♦ **Take the help.** Last, the one that is the most difficult for me, and I suspect many of us: Always take help when it's offered—whether you need it or not. Oof. Not an easy thing, especially for those of us who like to think of ourselves as strong, independent, and capable—Pitta. Yes, we are. And, observe your breath for a moment. There's an in breath; there's an out breath. It's what creates balance. Energy comes in; energy goes out. Maybe, for that time when we think we don't need help when it's offered, it will leave us a little extra energy to help out the next time someone needs us. Besides, you know how good it feels when you do something helpful for someone! Why would you rob someone else of the opportunity to feel good? Take the help.

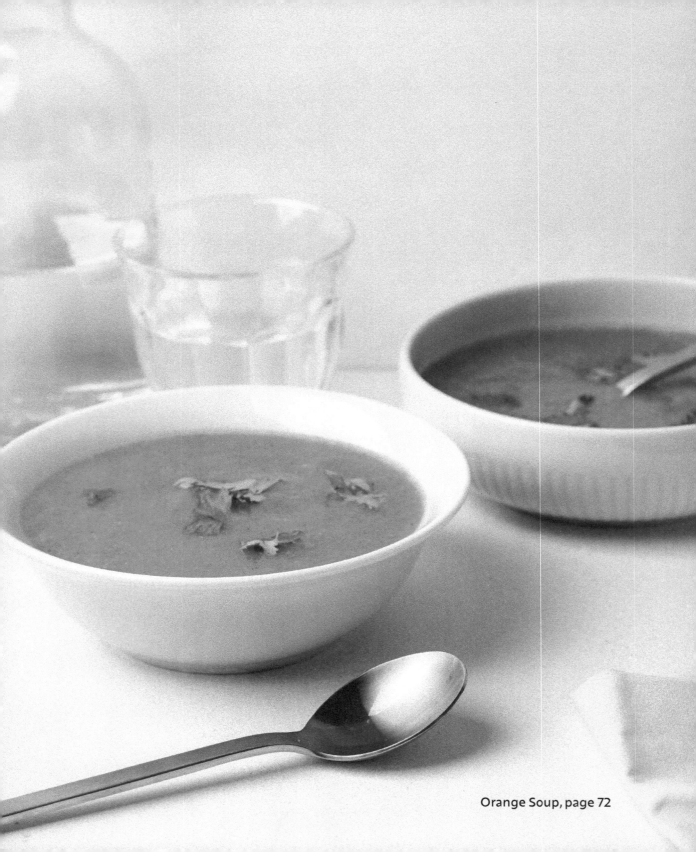

Orange Soup, page 72

6
KAPHA 7-DAY KICKSTART PLAN

All right, Kapha people, let's take stock of what's been going on. If you've been eating too much sugar or heavy food, letting your house get messy or cluttered, or just feel like you need a big reset to clear some space and make some changes, I got you! Here's your weeklong plan to start shifting some of that muddy energy. This plan will give you a good, thorough spring clean for your body, mind, and spirit. It is a perfect ritual for the spring equinox or anytime you're feeling slow, sluggish, heavy, mildly depressed, very uninspired—or all of the above! Try to schedule this so the last two days fall on nonworking days.

It's okay if there is resistance at first. Kapha types often have trouble getting started, but once that hurdle is jumped, your famous Kapha stamina and strength will take over. Perhaps you saw the title of this chapter and thought, "Yeah, I'll get around to that, I fully intend to do that . . . someday . . . ." That's all the more reason to do it *now*. I am here to give you a step stool to get over that hurdle. Just follow the directions. That's all you have to do. Trust that the rewards will begin to show themselves immediately. Ready? No? Yes. You are. You really are.

Bonus: Because Kapha people work so well with others and love company, you might want to enroll a friend to do this kickstart with you. You can help hold each other accountable and keep each other company. No quitting! See it through, even if you don't get to all of it.

Pregame Warm-up

Try not to do the whole "night-before-debauchery" thing. In other words, this cleanse will not be so strict that you feel deprived, so there is no need to go crazy the night before and eat a pizza or a gallon of ice cream, which will just have you waking up feeling uninspired and heavy. The night before you start, have dinner as usual and try to get to bed before 11:00 p.m. Leave your peppermint or eucalyptus oil and seven cotton pads on your nightstand before you go to sleep.

I recommend you get the following items:

- ◆ Body brush (with a long handle)
- ◆ Cotton pads, such as those used for makeup removal (1 bag)
- ◆ Epsom salts (1 large bag)
- ◆ Essential oils (citrus and either peppermint or eucalyptus)
- ◆ Journal
- ◆ Neti pot (ceramic, not plastic)
- ◆ Smudge stick (a bundle of herbs—traditionally white sage—used for cleansing purposes; see resources, page 158)
- ◆ Tongue scraper (copper if possible)

Grocery List

- Baking soda
- Bay leaves, dried
- Black mustard seeds
- Black peppercorns, whole
- Burdock root tea bags
- Chai tea bags, organic
- Chickpeas, dried
- Cinnamon, ground
- Cloves, whole
- Cumin seeds
- Extra-virgin olive oil
- Garlic (1 head)
- Garlic powder
- Ginger root, small knob
- Ginger, ground
- Grapefruit (1)
- Honey, raw organic
- Millet or basmati rice (1 pound)
- Paprika, ground
- Sea salt
- Turmeric, ground
- White vinegar

DAY 1
A New Morning

Get up 30 minutes earlier than usual, and don't hit the snooze button. If you've been getting up at 8:00 a.m., make it 7:30 a.m. If you've been getting up at 7:00 a.m., make it 6:30 a.m. Remember, you are in this for the long-term shifts, and if you make too drastic of a shift, it's unsettling and stressful for your body and mind. Your goal is to avoid stress with small, lasting changes.

Before you go anywhere, reach over to your nightstand and grab your bottle of peppermint or eucalyptus essential oil and a cotton pad. Pour two drops of the essential oil on the cotton pad. Cup the pad in front of your face, and take a deep breath. The scent will go from your olfactory nerve into your limbic brain very quickly, and you should feel more awake within seconds. Keep it with you to tuck into your pocket when you get dressed, if you wish.

Head to the bathroom. Relieve yourself, and then splash cold water on to your face. Scrape your tongue, brush your teeth, and use the neti pot.

NETI POTS

Neti pots are a great way to clear out the nasal passages—the air we breathe isn't always the cleanest, or we may be in an area where there is a lot of pollen, pet dander, or any of the other things that can provoke congestion. If you've never used one before, they can be a little tricky at first, so give yourself a few times with it if it does not go well immediately. Fill your neti pot about three-quarters of the way full with purified, room-temperature or slightly warmed water.

Add a pinch of sea salt (make sure it's just a pinch, or it will burn), and swirl to combine. Lean over a sink and tip your head to the left, gently inserting the spout into your right nostril. Not too far in! Let half the water slowly pour into your right nostril; it will clear away impurities as it comes out of the left side. You will need to breathe through your mouth as you do this. Then do the same for the left nostril. It might get a little drippy, so give your nose a good blow afterward.

1. Before breakfast, get outside and take a brisk 15- to 20-minute walk. If it's too cold outside, roll out your yoga mat and do the Kapha yoga routine on page 42.

2. When you get home, put a couple drops of your eucalyptus or peppermint oil on your shower floor.

3. Take your body brush, and give yourself a thorough brushing with gentle, long strokes, always toward the heart.

4. Take your refreshing, scent-infused shower.

5. Have a dosha-appropriate breakfast from the Kapha food suggestions on page 62, and wash your dishes immediately afterward.

6. In the afternoon, make an appointment for a haircut on the sixth day of this plan. Try to get an appointment for 4:00 p.m.

7. If it's in your budget, make an appointment for a deep-tissue massage on the last day of this plan. If not, ask around and see if someone has a good massage therapist you might be able to barter with. Offer to walk a dog, babysit a child, update a website, whatever your skill may be. We can all use a little help in some way. Try to get an appointment for 4:00 p.m.

8. That's it! That's the only set of actions you need to do differently today. Otherwise, go about your day as usual.

A New Afternoon

1. Do all the Day One morning activities.
2. Put a large saucepan of water (at least 6 cups) on to boil. Once it's boiling, remove the pot from the heat and add 2 bags of chai tea and 2 bags of burdock root tea to it, then let it cool and steep for 15 minutes. Remove the tea bags and drink 1 cup of the tea with 1 teaspoon of honey poured in at the last moment before you drink it. Ayurveda does not recommend cooking honey, as it loses some of its medicinal properties. Pour the rest of the tea (without honey) into a water bottle that you can take with you to drink throughout the day.
3. Before you leave the house, put your citrus oil in your bag.
4. Have a dosha-appropriate lunch from the Kapha food suggestions on page 94.
5. Try to drink all the tea you brought before 4:00 p.m. at the latest, as chai does have a small amount of caffeine. If possible, add 1 teaspoon of honey again right before you drink it.
6. Make sure that, if you have a job where you are sitting a lot, you get up once an hour and stretch a little, jog in place, or do a few jumping jacks.
7. At 4:00 p.m., take a big inhale of your citrus oil.
8. After work, get home as quickly as possible (without rushing, though!). Change out of your work clothes, and go for a run. Or a bike ride. Or take a Zumba class. Just do something to get the sweat going and the circulation happening.

DAY 3
A New Evening

1. Do all the Day One morning activities.
2. Do all the Day Two afternoon activities.
3. When you get home from your post-work exercise, take a quick, hot shower. Get in the shower, throw your arms up, and turn slowly around once or twice, just to get the sweat off. When you get out, dry yourself briskly and put on some comfy clothes or pajamas.

4. Head into the kitchen and make a batch of Kapha Masala (see page 64), and whatever dosha-appropriate dinner you want, putting some masala in as you are cooking. Sprinkle masala over your food if you didn't cook.

5. After dinner, do a final e-mail check and then climb into bed by 10:00 p.m. Lights out at 10 o'clock. On the dot.

6. That's it. Sweet dreams.

DAY 4
A New Routine for Sacred Space

1. Do all the Day One morning activities.

2. Do all the Day Two afternoon activities.

3. Do all the Day Three evening activities.

4. Add to your day when you can: Do your laundry, or drop it off to be done.

5. Add to your day when you can: Clean out your bookshelves, and drop off books at the Salvation Army or Goodwill.

6. That's it. Helping others will make you feel good. And notice you can do both: Take care of yourself and help others. It doesn't have to be one or the other. I know you give so much! You can give to yourself as well.

DAY 5
A New Sense of Accomplishment

1. Do all the Day One morning activities, and put ½ pound of dried chickpeas in a bowl with water to soak for kichadi later.

2. Do all the Day Two afternoon activities.

3. Do all the Day Three evening activities.

4. Add to your day when you can: Take a steam bath, go to a sauna, or take a hot bath with Epsom salts. For the bath, place 1 cup of Epsom salts in a jar with a lid, and add 3 drops of your citrus oil and 2 drops of your peppermint or eucalyptus oil. Give the jar a good shake, and dump its contents into your bath. This may be done in place of post-work exercise

if time is short. Try to stay in the sauna, steam bath, or hot bath for 20 minutes.

5. Make the Erleichda (Lighten Up!) Kichadi (see page 58) for dinner. You will have enough for tomorrow as well.

6. After dinner, clean your kitchen. First take a "before" picture. Mop the floor, then wipe down the counters and shelves. Throw out any dishes or utensils that are stained, warped, cracked, or not used regularly. Go through the refrigerator, and throw out any stale food. Remove the rest of the items, and wash the shelves thoroughly. Take an "after" picture, and feel proud of yourself.

7. Journal for a few minutes before bed around this idea: "I can take care of others more effectively when I take care of myself."

8. Lights out by 10:00 p.m.

DAY 6
A New Perspective

Hopefully this is a day you're not working. Stick with what you've started; don't sleep in or eat "cheat meals" or anything like that. You are moving toward new habits, and you will not be thrown off.

1. Do all the Day One morning activities.

2. Do all the Day Two afternoon activities.

3. Do all the Day Three evening activities.

4. If you've been doing the same exercise routine each day, change it up. Try a class you've never tried before: the mini-trampoline class, the rowing class, or whatever the new trend is. Ask a Pitta friend if you're not sure. Look for your afternoon exercise to begin around 2:00 p.m. and be done by 3:00 p.m.

5. After your shower, have a quick snack. A grapefruit half with cinnamon or a green smoothie is a great option.

6. Get your hair cut. Don't be late to your appointment!

7. Back from your haircut, have a kichadi dinner and let yourself digest for about 15 minutes.

8. Then, it's cleaning time! Slowly, working one section at a time, start in on your closets. Open up all the closets and drawers, take some "before" pictures, and get to work. Throw out whatever is stained, is ripped, or hasn't been worn in a year or more. Don't second guess yourself. It will get easier as you go.

9. At 9:30 p.m., shut it down for the night. You have made major headway, whether you finished your closet or not! Go ahead and open all your drawers and closets, and grab a metal bowl or pot from the kitchen. Light your smudge stick until it flames, then gently blow it out until it's smoldering and smoking. Holding the bowl under the stick with one hand to catch any falling ash, gently wave your smudge stick over the open closets and drawers. While you're at it, smudge yourself. Starting at your feet, wave the smudge stick over you and up to your head, circle your head three times, and smudge back down. Then tap out the embers in the bowl. If necessary, run a tiny bit of water over them, but don't soak the stick too much—you can reuse it. Take your "after" pictures, and feel proud of yourself. Mission accomplished!

10. Journal for five minutes or so before bed. Reflect on how it felt to throw things out, to clear space. If it was difficult or you didn't do it, reflect on why.

11. Turn the lights out by 10:00 p.m., and set your alarm for 5:00 a.m. Yes, you read that right. Just this once. Again, this should be a day you're not working.

DAY 7
A New Sankalpa (Sacred Promise)

1. Wake at 5:00 a.m. It will probably not be that difficult, as this is before Kapha time. Grab your essential oil from the nightstand, and use as usual. Get out of bed, and go to the window. If it's early spring, it should still be dark outside. Even if it's cold, open the window just for a minute and breathe in the spring air for a moment or two. Breathe deeply and slowly. Close the window, and go about your usual morning routine, but do a longer walk or a longer yoga routine (i.e., longer breath exercises,

two more rounds of sun salutations, etc., or find a guided yoga class online; see resources on page 158).

2. Have a dosha-appropriate breakfast from the Kapha food suggestions on page 62. Put ½ cup of dried chickpeas in a bowl with water for soaking.

3. You should have the day off, so this is the day to clean out the rest of your home. Even if you have someone in to clean for you, do it anyway. Take a few "before" photos, and don't just clean. Go into the junk drawer and get rid of the odd menus, keys, and business cards you don't use. Empty the garbage, and scrub out the garbage can. Clean out your drains by pouring 1 cup of baking soda into the drain, then 1 cup white vinegar after that.

4. At noon, stop, take "after" pictures, and make kichadi. Eat a bowl of kichadi, do the dishes, and go for a gentle walk or bike ride outside afterward; get some fresh air.

5. Go get your massage! You've earned it! If you were not able to book a massage, go online and find a restorative yoga class. Do a restorative sequence for an hour.

6. Come back, take a bath with Epsom salts and essential oils, and have kichadi for dinner.

7. After dinner, journal for 30 minutes or so about this week. What was the most difficult part of it? What did you just plain refuse to do? What are the top-three things you think you could do on a regular basis? What is the number-one thing you vow to do every day? Ritualize your answer to that. Record yourself saying it on your phone, write it on a piece of paper or sticky note, and place it where you can see it every day.

8. Get into bed, place your left hand on your heart, your right hand on your belly, and take a few long, slow breaths. Give yourself a moment of gratitude for your breath, your body, and your willingness to commit to self-care and healing. Send your efforts out to the greater good. Sweet dreams. Happy spring!

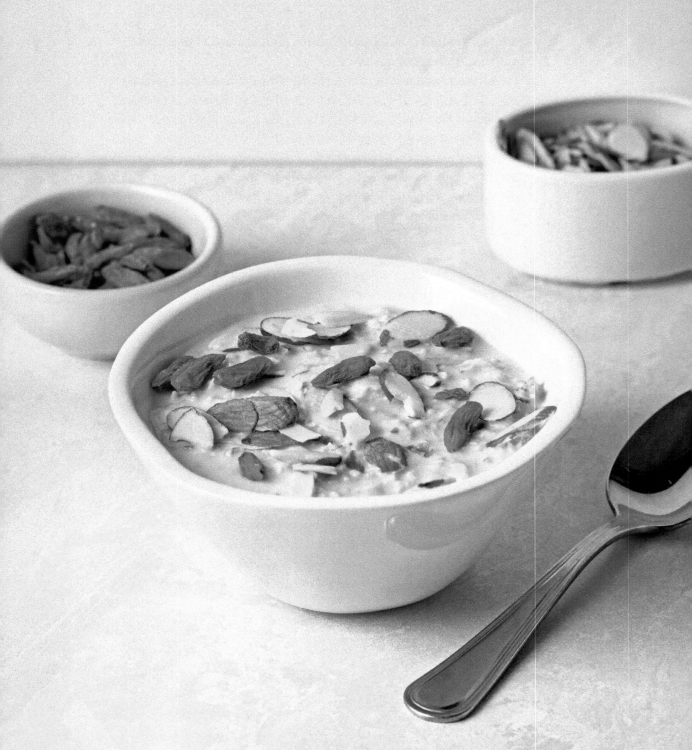

Overnight Oats, page 63

7

PITTA 7-DAY KICKSTART PLAN

Pitta folks, if you're headed toward burnout, take a full stop. Maybe you've been overdoing it at the gym, working too much and coming home hangry and wolfing down your food, or just feeling like lately you've been on the hamster wheel and can't stop running—I got you! Here is a clear, weeklong plan to make the Pitta fire more manageable. This time will give you a thorough refresh of your body, mind, and spirit. It is a perfect ritual for the last part of summer or anytime you're feeling like you're in danger of overheating in body and mind. Try to schedule this so the last two days fall on nonworking days.

It's time to jump off the aforementioned hamster wheel. The world will still keep going without you. You can take a break. It's okay if it is uncomfortable at first; it's hard for Pitta people to slow down and soften a bit. Trust that once you see how calm you feel and reflect on how that might help your efficiency, you will have your incentive to continue. And, seriously, don't you want to enjoy your life? Connect to people on a deeper level about things other than work? This is all to say, if you saw the title of this chapter and thought to yourself, "Yes, I will schedule that in, right after my trainer and spin class, my Apple stock hits $10,000, or my earnings season is over," then all the more reason to do it now. Learn to temper your fire so it's sustainable. Burnout wreaks havoc on you, your relationships, and your career. Slow down before you hit the wall! Remember, much of Ayurveda is preventive. Don't wait for the emergency.

Bonus: One of the best ways to balance Pitta is to remember to support others. You might want to enroll a friend to do this kickstart with you. You have to be honest with yourself, though; if it starts to feel like a competition with your friend and you have to "win," then forfeit. Yes. You read that right. Tell your friend they have won, you can't finish, and restart the plan on your own the following week without telling anyone.

Pregame Warm-up

The night before Day One, put your phone in your nightstand drawer instead of on your nightstand. It's still there if you absolutely must have it, and if you need the alarm to wake you up, you'll still be able to hear it. Call (not text or e-mail) a good friend, and make plans to have dinner on Day Four. Make an appointment for a massage around 4:00 p.m. on the last day of your kickstart. Check in with your doctor, and if it's deemed appropriate, make an appointment to donate blood early in the afternoon (around 2:00 p.m.) on the last day of this plan.

I recommend you get the following items:

- Essential oils (floral, such as rose, jasmine, or ylang ylang, and either peppermint or lime)
- Eye bag
- Journal
- Neti pot (ceramic, not plastic)
- Small bottle of organic fractionated coconut oil
- Tongue scraper (stainless steel)

Grocery List

- Almonds (4 ounces)
- Brown basmati rice (2 pounds)
- Cilantro (1 bunch)
- Coconut (1; if you can't find it, choose a dosha-appropriate fruit from the table on page 94)
- Coconut flakes, dried unsweetened (small bag)
- Coconut milk (1 [4-ounce] box or can)
- Coconut oil, organic and unrefined (1 [6-ounce] bottle)
- Coconut sugar (optional)
- Coconut water, raw (6 single servings)
- Coriander seeds
- Cucumbers, large (2)
- Cumin seeds
- Dates (small bag)
- Fennel seeds
- Ginger (1 [2-inch] piece)
- mung dal beans (1 pound)
- Saffron
- Sea salt
- Turmeric, ground
- Watermelon, small (1)
- White peppercorns, whole

"HOT" BLOOD

When I did *panchakarma* (a big Ayurvedic cleanse that can last anywhere from two weeks to a month) in Kerala, I had a pretty massive Pitta attack. It was awful. I got a massage with some medicated oil the first day, and within two days, my body was covered with eczema. My eyes, arms, and legs were itchy and uncomfortable, and I looked terrifying. One of the traditional therapies for excess Pitta is bloodletting. Sounds scary, but it's actually been a part of many traditional medicine practices. One of the locations of Pitta is in the blood, and when there's too much heat in the body, it can lead to various skin disorders. The idea behind this practice is that if the "hot" blood is taken away, the new blood that the body makes will be fresh, and the skin issues can subside. I was mildly nervous when the doctor in India said he was going to do it to me, but I trusted him completely. He stuck a needle in my arm and said, "Stop me when you feel faint." #wouldneverhappeninthe States. Sure enough, a minute or so in, I felt a little faint, he stopped, and over the next few days, the rash started to recede. His advice to me was to give blood once a year, as it was basically the same thing. Additionally, it is spiritually good for Pitta, as donating blood is an act of service.

DAY 1
Easing In

1. You probably already wake up pretty early, before 7:00 a.m. If not, move up your waking time by 30 minutes, setting an alarm if necessary. I doubt you're the "snooze" type, but if you are, skip the snooze and get up.

2. Go into the bathroom and brush your teeth, scrape your tongue (gently!), and use your neti pot (see page 118).

3. Take a shower, and add a few drops of the peppermint or lime essential oil to your bodywash, if you use that. If you use a bar of soap, just soap up a washcloth and add a couple drops of the oil to that.

4. Get dressed. Wear blue, green, gray, white, or purple—no red, yellow, or orange. And try to stick to natural fibers; your Pitta skin needs to breathe.

5. If this is the time you usually work out, do that and have breakfast afterward. If not, go right into breakfast.

6. Head into the kitchen and have a dosha-appropriate breakfast from the Pitta food suggestions on page 63. While you are eating, keep the phone away from you. Give yourself a tech break this week while you are eating. That goes for all three meals. I know. Just do it. If you drink coffee or tea in the morning, add some coconut milk to it.

7. Pack your work bag with some appropriate snacks. That could be some cut fresh watermelon, a small bag of almonds, a few pieces of fresh coconut, a couple of dates, etc. If you work out after work, add your workout clothes. Whatever your regular workout is today, do it as usual, drink coconut water afterward, and eat some fresh cucumber.

8. Before you leave your house, deeply inhale your floral oil, taking a full breath. Tuck the essential oil bottle into your bag. Grab the lime or peppermint oil from the bathroom as well.

9. Assuming you had lunch around noon or 1:00 p.m., have your snack around 4:00 p.m. When you finish your snack, inhale the floral, lime, or peppermint oil, whichever appeals to you.

10. Before bed, place your phone in your nightstand drawer, get your bottle of coconut oil and pour a palmful into your hand. Add a few drops of the floral oil, and rub it into your feet. It's very grounding and helpful for proper rest. Try to be in bed by 10:00 p.m. If that's not possible, make it 11:00 p.m. at the latest.

DAY 2
Water Cure

1. Do all the Day One morning activities.
2. During your workday, make a point of drinking extra water: Aim for 64 ounces a day. Even if you fall a little short, you'll still be well hydrated. Add fresh mint or a squeeze of lime to it, if you enjoy that. Peppermint and lime both support digestion. Peppermint is a little more drying; lime is a little more lubricating, so choose accordingly (i.e., if it's a very humid day, pick the peppermint; if it's a very dry day, pick the lime).
3. If you usually work out after work, skip it today. Go for a walk in nature instead. Even if you live in a city, find a nearby river, lake, or park. Bonus points for calling a friend or a date to come with you.
4. Double bonus points for inviting the friend or date home with you for dinner. Triple bonus points for cooking for them! If you are dining alone, give yourself an experience. Put the tech away (you promised!), and play some nice music and light a candle while you eat. Chew slowly and thoroughly.
5. After dinner, keep the music on and the tech off. Lie down on your couch on your left side for 10 minutes. Lying on your left side opens up your right breath channel, or what we call in yoga the *Pingala nadi*. This is helpful for proper digestion.
6. After, go online and find at least a 20-minute yoga nidra routine, pick a comfy and quiet place, and put the nidra recording on. Lie down on your back with a pillow or folded blanket under your head, and place an eye pillow over your eyes.
7. Give yourself a foot rub, and turn the lights out by 11:00 p.m. at the latest.

DAY 3
Body Temple

1. Do all the Day One morning activities.
2. Do all the Day Two afternoon activities, except that this can be a post-work workout day again. Switch it up, though. If this is a day you normally do a HIIT routine or spin class, try a yoga, tai chi, or qigong

class instead. Find something soothing for the nervous system and gentle on the body.

3. When you get home from class, put 1 cup of brown basmati rice and ½ cup of mung beans in a large bowl with water to soak, then take a quick shower.

4. Make the Cool-It-Down Kichadi (see page 59) for dinner, and sit down to enjoy your meal without phone, e-mail, or reading.

5. After dinner, go online and find a local charity looking for volunteers. Sign up to do some volunteer work for Day Six of this plan. If you cannot find something, volunteer to babysit a friend's kids, walk all the dogs in your neighborhood, or find something else that resonates with you. You can also plan to make a bunch of sandwiches to leave with the homeless around your community, clean out your closets for a big Goodwill drop-off, make phone calls for a cause, or clean an elderly person's house. But plan it. Make the commitment.

6. Listen to a guided meditation, check your e-mail, give yourself a foot massage, and get to sleep before 11:00 p.m.

DAY 4
Listen for Love

1. Do all the Day One morning activities.

2. Have leftover kichadi for breakfast and lunch, if you have leftovers. If not, have a dosha-appropriate breakfast and lunch from the Pitta food suggestions on page 94.

3. Make sure you are drinking water and using your oils.

4. After work, meet your friend you spoke with the night before you started for a catch-up dinner. If for some reason that doesn't happen, call an old friend you haven't seen in a while.

5. At dinner or after dinner at home on the phone, listen twice as much as you speak, and don't interrupt your friend. Even . . . when . . . they . . . talk . . . slowly.

6. Do yoga nidra, take a quick shower, put on your pajamas, and go to sleep before 11:00 p.m.

DAY 5
Speak for Love

1. Do all the Day One morning activities.

2. Make sure you are drinking water and using your oils.

3. Be impeccable with your word. Here's a big challenge for you. Yesterday you were working on your listening skills. Today, and for the next two days, you'll be working on your communication skills. Be mindful of your language, tone of voice, and pace of dialogue. Speaking to people in a way that makes them feel safe, not intimidated, is an important thing for Pitta people. I invite you to take the words *kickass*, *badass*, *hardcore*, *slay*, and *killing it*, out of your vocabulary today. Don't rely on curse words to get your point across or to be provocative. Put a jar on your counter, and use it to count up how many times during the day you speak in a way that is violent, profane, or intimidating, adding a dollar to the jar each time. At the end of the week, donate the money to your favorite cause.

4. After work, try another new fitness class. Try a dance class of some sort, whether it's Zumba, hip-hop, or salsa. Something with music and people and fun—even if you feel a little dumb at first. Get out there and laugh at yourself! Exercise can be fun and social, not just relentless.

5. When you get home from work, skip Netflix, Hulu, and YouTube. Instead, go online and find a 10-minute loving-kindness guided meditation.

6. Make Cool-It-Down Kichadi (see page 59) for dinner, and after dinner, journal about your communication skills. Was it hard to slow down when you spoke? Did you feel like you didn't have enough oomph in your conversations to make them exciting today? Were you able to speak in a way that people could feel like your equals instead of your inferiors? How often do you think you have done that in the past?

7. Lights out by 11:00 p.m. at the latest.

Selfless Service

1. Hopefully this is a day off for you. Do all the Day One morning activities.
2. Make sure you are drinking water and using your oils.
3. You're off to make a difference. It's your volunteer day or day of service. Do this the entire day, the same amount of time you would normally spend at work. If it feels like too much, think about it. Why is it okay when it's work?
4. At the end of the day, journal about your day. How did it feel to be of service? Did it help you appreciate the blessings in your life? Is it something you could see yourself doing on a regular basis? How often? Could you commit to a full day, or is a half day more realistic?
5. Lights out by 11:00 p.m. at the latest. Job well done! Sleep well!

Pamper Me

1. Sleep in. Ignore your alarm. When you wake up, linger in bed for a little while. If you have a partner, make love! Yes, if you must brush your teeth and scrape your tongue first, that's fine. But then get right back into bed and snuggle up. Initiate with your partner, and if they aren't in the mood, give them a back rub or make them breakfast instead.
2. Take a long, luxurious bath. Put a few drops of your essential oils into your bodywash, and put some of the bodywash in the bathwater while you soak. Add ½ cup of coconut milk, and turn your bath into a yummy spa.
3. After your bath, go for a long walk. Smile at three people along the way—a big, genuine grin.
4. Buy yourself some flowers on the way back.
5. Either take yourself out to lunch or have a luxurious lunch at home, whatever that means to you. It could mean having an appetizer, main course, and dessert, or maybe it means buying the fancy burrata cheese or expensive gelato at the supermarket. Eat something that feels like a celebration.

6. After your lunch, leave the dishes. Yes, I said leave the dishes. You can do them later. You don't need to be perfect.

7. If it's nice out, go back outside with a book you've been meaning to read. Find a bench or a tree or a soft lawn to read on. Spend an hour reading. No texting. If you don't have a book to read, call an old friend and chat.

8. If you are going to donate blood, do it now.

9. Go to your massage. You've earned it! If you donated blood, wait at least a couple of hours, and make sure you tell your body worker that you have done it so they can avoid your arm and be more gentle. If a massage is not in the budget, go to a restorative yoga class.

10. Come home from the massage and make a quiet dinner. Do all the dishes from lunch and dinner, and clean the kitchen.

11. Do the loving-kindness meditation from Day Five again after dinner.

12. Quickly check e-mail, then journal about your week. What worked for you? What didn't? What surprised you about yourself? Do you feel your relationships improved this week? Why is that important?

13. Lights out by 11:00 p.m. at the latest. Congratulations! You did it!

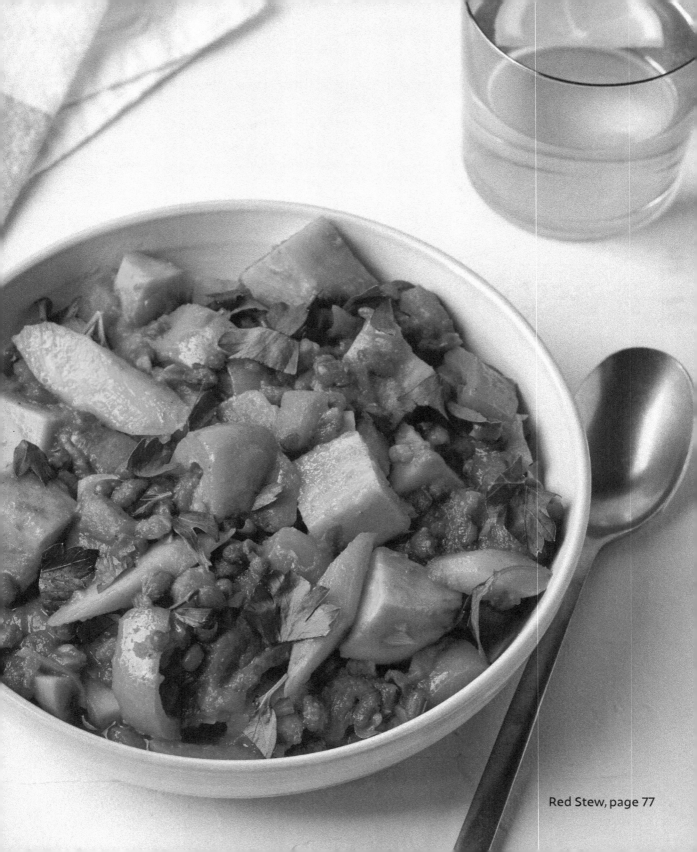

Red Stew, page 77

8
VATA 7-DAY KICKSTART PLAN

Vata people, I get it. I've been there. You're doing too much or you're traveling too much, and proper nutrition and sleep hasn't been happening. Now your body is starting to break down. Your nervous system is on continuous high alert, your immunity sucks, and you're feeling alarmingly depleted. All of a sudden, the screech of subway brakes or a wailing baby (even if they're your own!) makes you hold your ears and cringe. Let's do something about it. We will take it slow and steady, and at the end of the week, I think you will be sleeping better and feeling less frantic and more grounded. Let's take some actions to get you feeling less overwhelmed and more empowered. A good time to do this plan is around the second week of November (especially if you're gearing up for a holiday season), or anytime you feel like your stress is high and your immunity is low.

Pregame Warm-up

Get yourself in this mind-set. For the next week, you are like an infant. You need to be nourished, safe, and swaddled in self-care. The night before you start, set up a cozy dinner at your place with a few friends for Day Five. Make sure to be in bed by 10:00 p.m. at the latest. You will sleep a lot better and wake up ready to make some changes. Make sure your bedroom is dark, quiet, and cozy, and power down all your electronics by 9:00 p.m. Place a journal and pen on your nightstand before you go to sleep.

I suggest you get the following items:

- Carrier oil, preferably sesame (1 bottle)
- Epsom salts (1 large bag)
- Essential oils (lavender or geranium, and an immunity blend that includes at least two of the following oils: rosemary, lemon, wild orange, tea tree, clove, cinnamon, ginger)
- Journal
- Neti pot (ceramic, not plastic)
- Tongue scraper
- Triphala powder

Grocery List

- Almond butter (1 jar) or vegan protein powder
- Avocados (3)
- Bay leaves, dried
- Black peppercorns, whole, or freshly ground black pepper
- Bread, whole-grain, sprouted, organic, or gluten-free (1 loaf)
- Brown basmati rice (2 pounds)
- Butter, unsalted, organic (1 pound) or organic sesame oil
- Cilantro (1 bunch)
- Cinnamon sticks (2 [3-inch])
- Cloves, whole
- Coconut, unsweetened shredded
- Coriander seeds
- Cumin seeds
- Ginger, (1 [3-inch]) piece
- Green cardamom pods
- Hummus, high-quality (1 package) or homemade (see page 68)
- Lemons (2)
- Sea salt
- Sesame seeds
- Split mung beans (2 pounds)
- Split mung dal (1 pound)
- Sweet potatoes, large (4)
- Tulsi tea bags, any flavor you wish
- Turmeric, ground
- Yellow mustard seeds

New Beginning

1. Wake up early; around 5:30 a.m. is ideal. If it's later, that's okay, but try to have at least an hour and a half before you need to leave the house. Grab your pen and journal off your nightstand, and write about how you slept. Include any dreams you remember. Record whether you got up during the night. If you did, were you able to go back to sleep quickly/slowly/not at all? Then do a page of stream-of-consciousness writing. Get in touch with your unconscious and creative side right away.

2. Go to your bathroom, brush your teeth, scrape your tongue, and use the neti pot (see page 118 for instructions). Put a little sesame oil on your pinky finger, and roll it around in each nostril for lubrication after you use your neti pot. Wash your hands, and then do the same thing for your ear—place sesame oil on your pinkies and do a gentle, lubricating swirl.

3. Head to the kitchen and make warm water, at least 16 ounces. Quarter one of the lemons, and squeeze it into the water. Drink at least half right away.

4. Do the Vata yoga routine (see page 46), or bundle up and go for a walk for 20 minutes. Leave your headphones at home; it's too distracting. You want to feel as present and grounded as possible right now. Be mindful of your feet on the ground and the environment around you.

5. Have a dosha-appropriate breakfast from the Vata food suggestions on page 63.

6. After breakfast, clean up the kitchen.

7. Finally, finish your water and put your immunity oil in your bag to take with you. During the day, inhale the blend and breathe the scent in deeply.

8. Turn the lights out by 10:00 p.m. Even if you don't think you will be able to sleep, do it anyway.

9. That's all you need to do the first day. You don't want to get overwhelmed! It's so important for you to practice taking things slowly.

Home Spa

1. Do all the morning activities from Day One. Notice whether your sleep pattern has changed. Pack your tulsi tea to take with you.

2. During the day, make a conscious effort to have two cups of tulsi tea, and have a dosha-appropriate lunch from the Vata food suggestions on page 94.

3. When you get home from work at night, take a bath. Combine 1 drop of your immunity oil, 4 drops of your floral oil, and 1 cup of Epsom salts in a glass jar. Cover it, and give it a good shake. Add the salts to your bathwater. If you don't have a bathtub, take a long, leisurely shower instead. Make sure the water isn't too hot, though, as that will dry you out even more.

4. After your bath or shower, get your bottle of sesame oil and give yourself a rubdown with that. You can put a couple drops of lavender or geranium in a palmful of oil. Starting at your feet, gently rub oil into yourself, all the way up to your neck.

5. Put on pajamas that feel soft and warm.

6. Add ½ teaspoon of triphala to 1 cup of warm water, and drink it before bed.

7. Get into bed and listen to a guided meditation for sleep, or do your own quiet meditation. Turn the lights out by 10:00 p.m., if possible. Sweet dreams!

Grounding 101

1. Do all the Day One morning activities.
2. Do all the Day Two afternoon activities.
3. When you get home from work, put 1 cup of split mung dal in water to soak.
4. It's probably been a few hours since you had lunch. Have a snack while you are soaking the beans: A slice of toast with either almond butter, hummus, or avocado makes a lovely snack with a good mix of fiber and healthy fats.
5. Get two pillows and a blanket from your room. Find a quiet corner. Set an alarm on your phone to a tone that isn't jarring when it goes off. Put the timer on for 20 minutes. Fold your blanket into quarters. This will be your pillow for your head. Lie down with your blanket pillow under your head, and then come into Reclining Goddess (see page 43, E) pose with a pillow under each thigh for support. Close your eyes, put both hands on your belly, and feel your breath. If you fall asleep, it's fine. It just means you needed to rest.
6. When the timer goes off, try not to bolt out of the pose. Slowly bring your knees together and roll onto your right side, then use your arms to come up to sit. Sit cross-legged or come to sit on your heels on your blanket, if that feels better. Place just the fingertips of your right hand on the ground. With your left hand, have the index finger touching the first knuckle of your thumb. This is called Bhumisparsha mudra, and it means "Gesture of Touching the Earth." It's a reminder that in the midst of everything, we can be still and connect to our roots. Stay there as long as you wish, preferably 10 minutes or so.
7. When you're done, take a shower, give yourself an oil rubdown, and go into the kitchen to make Bring-Me-Back Kichadi (see page 60).
8. Eat your dinner (no phone or computer while you eat), clean up after, and then take your journal and get into bed.
9. Write about your day. Were you feeling less frantic? What was your experience of the restorative yoga pose and the mudra meditation? Did you feel more present for your meal?
10. Lights out by 10:00 p.m. again, if possible.

I strongly encourage all of the dosha types to find a good restorative yoga class. Vata people, you would benefit from taking it once a week, Pitta people twice a month, and Kapha people once a month. Here's what I have noticed when I teach restorative yoga. People are unsure exactly how to set themselves up well, and will settle for "Well, it feels okay, so I will just make do." Three minutes into it and their nervous system is still on high alert, and they are getting fidgety. One of my restorative teachers used to say that, when setting up a restorative yoga pose, we should be very "princess and the pea" about it—meaning, if a prop is just slightly off, it actually makes a huge difference. Restorative yoga should feel amazing, and if it doesn't, your setup is a little off. Please speak up! Let the teacher know if the pose is bothering your lower back, knee, shoulder, etc., right away so they can help you with the setup or find a different pose for you.

DAY 4
The Slow Down

1. Do all the Day One morning activities.
2. Going into work, I have a challenge for you. Notice all the times you rush—to the subway, to catch the elevator, to get your lunch. Perhaps you eat in a rush, or even speak in a rush—slow down! Work on being mindful of time management. Maybe you wouldn't have to rush to work if you left yourself more time. Maybe you wouldn't have to gulp your food if you were stricter with yourself about not getting sidetracked with whatever you're working on before lunch. And last, you don't have to get all the words out in one breath. Linger, and let what you say land in your conversations. Even if you're excited. Because, let's face it, most of the time, you're excited. So, it's a good idea to learn how to manage yourself within the excitement.
3. Have leftover kichadi for lunch.
4. After work, find some sort of body-mind exercise class. Something calming, strengthening, and not too fast. Skip the latest HIIT class; instead, look for a tai chi, yoga, qigong, or Pilates class. If you can't find one, go home and look one up online, and spend at least 45 minutes doing it.

5. Put split mung dal in to soak for Bring-Me-Back Kichadi (see page 60). Yes, again. You're creating healthy habits to replace the habits that are already there, like skipping meals or grabbing whatever is nearby.

6. While the beans are soaking, make ghee if you chose to get the butter. Add the pound of unsalted butter to a saucepan, and bring it to a gentle boil. Skim off the foam that collects, and keep doing that until the butter is clear. When it is all clear, let it cool and carefully pour it into a glass jar. Use the ghee for your kichadi base, and add an extra teaspoon of ghee on top of your portion when you are finished.

7. After dinner and cleanup, make yourself a cup of Golden Milk (see page 91).

8. Get into bed, slowly sip your milk, and write in your journal. How did it feel to slow down? When you didn't slow down, do you know why? Was your time today used effectively?

9. Turn the lights out by 10:00 p.m.

WAIT YOUR TURN

I used to take meditation workshops with a wonderful Buddhist meditation teacher. She had been teaching for around 30 years, and had been meditating even longer. We ended up being friends, and we would go out sometimes to hear music together. Having a conversation with her was a very different experience for me. There was so much space in the conversation, because she considered her words and choices carefully. I would fidget and want to "help her" make a decision or a point. And something in me knew to just stay quiet and learn to relax into it. To be honest, I have a tendency to interrupt people—maybe you can relate? It's a terrible habit. Sometimes it comes from a good place (e.g., "I am so into this conversation, I am paying such fervent attention, I know exactly what you're going to say"). And then I butt in on what someone is telling me. Here's the thing: You don't actually know what someone else is going to say, and interrupting is rude. I have been working on this one for a while now, and I'm proud to say I'm better at it. And if it does happen, I quickly apologize and say, "Please go on." My Vata peeps, if it seems like the conversation is too slow and you catch yourself trying to speed it up, stop. Breathe. Drop into your body. And wait for your opening.

DAY 5

Community Is the Guru

1. Do all the Day One morning activities. Stick with the slower pace.
2. Do all the Day Two afternoon activities. Stick with the slower pace.
3. Have leftover kichadi for lunch.
4. This is the day for your dinner with friends, so if you need to send a few text reminders during the day, do that.
5. On your way home from work, if it's in your budget, pick up some flowers for a pretty table arrangement. If you like to have wine occasionally, and you know your friends might enjoy that, get a bottle of wine.
6. When you get home, make up a side dish of Veggie Stir-Fry (see page 70) and the kichadi. Light some candles for the table, if you have them.
7. Sit down to a lovely Ayurvedic dinner with your friends. You can even make them Golden Milk (see page 91) after dinner! Talk, laugh, sympathize, and be with each other. It's such good medicine!
8. Get your friends to help you clean up.
9. To 1 cup of warm water, add ½ teaspoon of triphala, and drink it before bed. Hopefully, tomorrow is a day off so you can sleep in if you got to bed a little later tonight.
10. Before you sleep, send some prayers out to your friends, your family, and your loved ones. Energetically connect to them and feel the warmth of connection. You love, and you are loved. Smile into feeling that as you drift to sleep.

DAY 6

Silence Is Golden

1. Today will be a day of vocal rest for you. In yoga, we call this the practice of mauna. Talking takes energy, and Vata people like to chatter. See if you can make this a day of no talking or even texting until sunset.
2. Do your morning activities, and then take part of the day to organize your living space. Go through old mail, and make piles of what can be thrown out and what needs further attention. Clean out your junk

drawer and/or desk. Go through your bookshelf, and make a stack of books you can let go of to bring to your local charity. Go through your computer and clean up your files. Clear your information channels.

3. When you get hungry, have some leftover kichadi or a dosha-appropriate lunch from the Vata food suggestions on page 94.

4. After lunch, go through your e-mails. Delete what needs to be deleted, empty your spam folder, and set up your calendar for the next month. You won't get to all of it, but make some headway for a half hour or so. Try to stay off social media, it ends up sucking us in for too long. Set a limit of one hour to deal with correspondence.

5. When you're done, go for another walk outside. Yes, even if it's cold. Bundle up well. Try to get to someplace you can see trees, water, or both. Spend an hour outside. Watch the sunset. Don't purchase anything on your walk.

6. When you return, have a cup of tulsi tea and breathe in your immunity formula essential oil.

7. You might find that you actually don't want to speak after sunset. If that is the case, honor that. Send any texts that you feel are necessary. If you do wish to speak, try to keep the "silent" energy by making your voice soft, slow, and gentle.

8. Have a dosha-appropriate soupy dinner (see pages 76 and 77) on the early side. Clean up, and head to the bathroom for a shower or bath.

9. Post shower or bath, do an oil rubdown with sesame oil, climb into bed, and journal for a few minutes on how it felt to be silent today. Did it make you feel replenished? Or did it feel like a punishment? If so, why? Vow to take a silent day once a month. You can find one day.

10. Lights out by 9:30 p.m. tonight. It's the last night of your kickstart, and you have been detoxing big time. Give your body the extra rest it needs. Set your alarm for 5:30 a.m. again.

DAY 7
Filling the Well

1. Do all the Day One morning activities.
2. After breakfast, catch up on any e-mails or phone calls you need to get to, then get dressed (make sure you wear comfy shoes) and pack your oils and books that you plan to donate.
3. Take today as a "refill" day. Linger in a museum, or go see a documentary or new movie you've heard good things about. Find a pottery class or a lecture to attend. Take some photos of things you see that resonate with you.
4. Have a hearty lunch out, and then do your grocery shopping for the week so you feel prepared.
5. When you get home, do your laundry and any cleaning that needs to be done.
6. At sunset, do your Restorative Goddess pose and mudra meditation (see page 139, #5 and #6).
7. Make dinner, eat, and then call one of your besties and have a good heart-to-heart.
8. When you get off the phone, journal about your day. Was there anything you saw or did that was particularly inspiring? Is there some creative expression in you that feels sparked, whether it's writing a poem, a blog, or a long letter? Or is there a picture to paint or a play to write or a song to compose? And then move on to your week. What was easy? What wasn't? What do you think you will continue to do? Was there anything you simply refused to do, and why?
9. You had a week of self-care, community, creativity, and clarity. It's all there. Send yourself some love and appreciation, and then lights out. Sweet dreams.

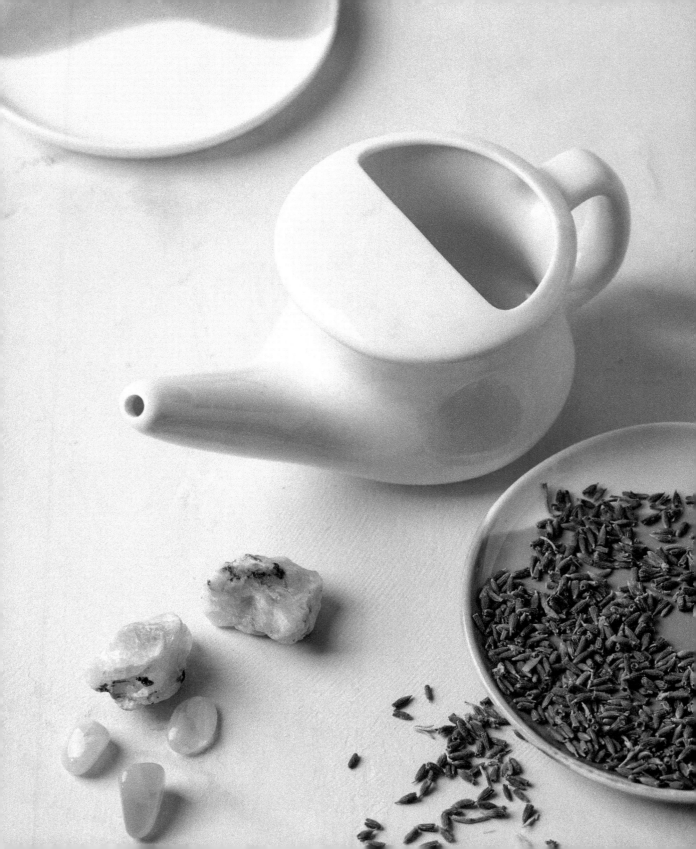

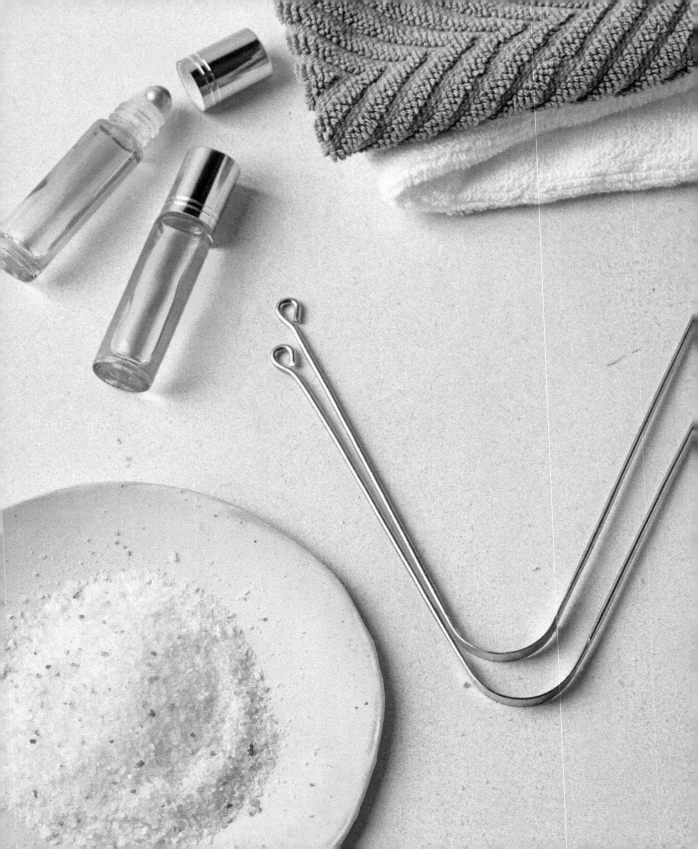

9

AYURVEDA
EVERY DAY

Congratulations! You have made it through your weeklong
kickstart! Thank you so much for trusting this process.
Thank you for having the willingness to make changes.
Thank you for helping keep the science of Ayurveda alive!
Seven days is such a great beginning. So . . . now what?

How Did That Feel?

Just for today, what feels sustainable from your week and what doesn't? It's helpful to go back and read your journal entries. Write down three things from your week that you think you could keep up with on a regular basis, whether it is every day, once a week, or once a month.

1. ....
2. ....
3. ....

Next, take note of how you felt on the day you actually managed to do most of the suggested actions. Give yourself a pat on the back. Really! We all need some encouragement and validation when we have made a breakthrough, whether it is big or small. Take a moment and vow to yourself to stay with those three actions you chose, and little by little, you can keep adding to them with other positive habits. Because really, what is the alternative? Sure, you could keep things exactly as they are and, at some point, be forced into a complete stop. But you're in a different place now. So why do that? You have a big, beautiful life to lead, you have important work to do, and you have people who depend on you. Ruining your health is letting yourself (and others) down.

Change Is Absolutely Possible

To get the point across when I teach workshops and trainings, I often describe an old-fashioned gadget called a Newton's cradle. You might've seen one at some point—it's a wooden frame, with 20 or so strings hanging down. All the strings have metal balls at the end of them. If you pull one of the balls at one end high up away from the others and let it go, it hits the other balls and the ball at the far side swings up. That ball returns to hit the balls closest to it until the original side again lifts and crashes back down—this goes on with less and less of a swing until the balls once again land quietly in the middle.

The way I see it, that's how most of us deal with imbalance in our lives. We skip sleep and work too much (first ball), and after we become exhausted and feel heavy, we drink a big espresso (last ball) to feel light. But then we feel spastic so we have some extra wine with dinner (first ball) and then feel heavy and pass out only to wake up super late in the morning feeling terrible. So we pop a bunch of medicine (last ball) to feel light again so we can work too much and skip sleep (again, first ball), and so on and so on. But here's the thing: If we never get too light/exhausted/ungrounded, then we never have to reach for extreme measures (excess in food/caffeine/stuff) to feel balanced. If we never get too overheated/ inflamed/aggressive, then we never have to reach for extreme measures (ice baths/rigid diets/anger management classes) to feel balanced. If we never get too oily/slow/foggy, we never have to reach for extreme measures (multiple daily hot yoga classes/energy drinks/overpriced supplements) to feel balanced.

Modern Ayurveda offers us another way. Instead of wildly swinging from one side to another, how about we hang out in the middle a little longer? It's so much more efficient with our physical and mental energy! Hopefully, the kickstarts gave you a deeper understanding of how the right actions for you can be incorporated into your life, and if you didn't get to all of them, no worries—you have more to look forward to. Try to incorporate the actions you didn't get to when you feel that some of your new practices have become habits. It's an ever-evolving way of being, and isn't that the good life: small daily actions that add up to a whole program of self-care?

If You Do Anything, Do This

All in all, I truly think the best approach these days is kinder, gentler, and more sustainable. Self-care should never feel restrictive or punishing—it should be a gift you give yourself on a daily basis. And sure, there will still be times when the ecosystem of your life gets in the way and you once again find yourself out of balance. Contemplate this: It's never really self-sabotage. It's a combination of what life throws at you and how you have learned to cope with it. Pretty much everything you do that you keep beating yourself up about—you're still smoking, working too much, drinking too much, or eating unhealthily—has served you at some point. It temporarily made the issue go away, and made you feel better in the moment. Let's forgive ourselves these missteps, and take them as part of a deeper understanding of what not to do.

Remember in school when you got homework? Well, here's some homework for life. Yeah. Because that's the truth of it. Balance is a dynamic state. It's not fixed. It's a constant juggling act, and you can either practice that and get adept, or drop the ball(s) and slink away. You've chosen to get adept. Great! It takes practice, commitment, acceptance, and ease. The approach you take to getting balanced has to be balanced as well! In a culture that talks about work as a "grind," how do we modernize this middle way?

Through understanding and follow-through. Modern Ayurveda can be applied to your life, either in a big way or a small way, on a daily basis. You can come to see that it is not just what you eat, what you drink, or what yoga poses are good for you. It's also the way you think and look at *all* of your decisions and actions. Are your choices leading you closer to health and happiness, or taking you further away? I want to get closer—and clearly, so do you, as you've made it to the last chapter.

Now that you have a greater understanding of yourself, you can start to think in a way that feels like preventive care. Here's a quick review.

Kapha people, you naturally have the qualities of heavy, oily, slow, and cold in body and mind. You need to think of all of your choices as ones that associate with the qualities of light, dry, fast, and hot for you to keep balance. Your top three daily balancers should be:

1. Move your body enough to sweat.
2. Stay away from too much heavy food.
3. Have less stuff! For every one thing you bring into your home, get rid of two things.

Pitta people, you naturally have the qualities of hot, light, oily, and fast in body and mind. You need to think of all of your choices as ones that associate with the qualities of cool, heavy, dry, and slow for you to keep balance. Your top three daily balancers should be:

1. Embrace water—drink it, swim in it, bathe in it, walk by it.
2. Stay away from too much spicy food.
3. Look for a way to be of service every day (e.g., volunteer your time, money, energy, or expertise to someone who needs it).

Vata people, you naturally have the qualities of cold, dry, light, and fast in body and mind. You need to think of all of your choices as ones that associate with the qualities of warm, oily, heavy, and slow for you to keep balance. Your top three daily balancers should be

1. Slow down! Move, talk, and eat more slowly.
2. Make sure you are eating regularly; no skipping meals.
3. Massage your feet nightly with a base of sesame oil and some grounding essential oils, such as cedarwood.

See how these balancers can apply to life. Taking a sweater along in case you get cold is a choice, and if you understand that cold is what you already have and therefore don't need, it's no longer a "choice." Choosing to add more oil to your meal is a choice, and if you understand that too much oil is not good for you, it's no longer a choice. Choosing to take a vacation in Arizona is a choice, and if you understand—well, you get it. And hopefully all those "non-choice" actions start to look like a lifetime plan of self-care that becomes second nature, just a part of who you are and what you do. If you feel like there are days that you need more inspiration to keep making non-choices, reread your journal from your kickstart week. Or do another kickstart. Maybe you'll be more willing to try the parts you skipped this time. Let it all evolve. Slow and steady.

EVERY DAY

I remember being at a birthday party a bunch of years ago where they brought out a big, sugary birthday cake with strawberries. I had been eating more Ayurvedically and didn't want it, not even a taste. When a plate came around to me, I said, "None for me, thanks." Someone at the party said, "Just have a slice. You know you want it." And I said, "Actually, I don't," and smiled and passed the plate down. And it was true. In the same way, I've weaned myself off hot sauce. You can get to a point where the stuff that doesn't serve you is not at all interesting. It's a process. As I've said, there are still times when it feels like a choice to me, and I make a not-so-good one. I have learned to be happy for the progress I have made, and I try to be gently encouraging with myself around the areas where I still have work to do. We are all in it together! You are now a part of the Ayurvedic community and lineage. We are millions (and millions) strong!

I took a great yoga workshop once where the teacher, Rod Stryker, was talking about the yoga world these days. He said, "People are always coming out with the newest, latest yoga style. They say it is amazing, revolutionary, and completely original. My thought is, 'If it's that good, why hasn't anyone done it before?'" Bam. Mic drop.

This applies to health as well. Come on, which system would you want to base your precious well-being on? One that has four—or even 40—years of research, development, and testing, or one that has four thousand years of research, development, and testing? Ayurveda has withstood the test of time. Enough people in enough places for thousands of years have benefited so much from its principles and practices that they passed it on, taught it to their communities and families, and shared it with the West and around the world. It has worked its way into cooking schools, wellness websites, and yoga centers. There have been rave reviews in blogs, videos, and social media. Hey, it made its way to *you* and got you to pick up this book. If it resonated with you and got you to shift a few daily actions and feel better in body and mind, then it has done its job. Pass it on!

I'm so honored to have been able to share this work with you. May your self-care and understanding keep you well for your family, loved ones, and community. May it keep you in an abundance of health that allows you to do the work you are meant to do in this world. Find a way to use that work to serve all, and I can promise you a lifetime of true joy.

Namaste,
Ali

Index

Resources

Recommended Reading

Miller, Light, and Bryan Miller. *Ayurveda & Aromatherapy: The Earth Essential Guide to Ancient Wisdom and Modern Healing*. Twin Lakes: Lotus Press, 1996.

Morningstar, Amadea, and Urmila Desai. *The Ayurvedic Cookbook*. Twin Lakes: Lotus Press, 1992.

Sachs, Melanie. *Ayurvedic Beauty Care: Ageless Techniques to Invoke Natural Beauty*. Twin Lakes: Lotus Press, 1994.

Welch, Claudia. *Balance Your Hormones, Balance Your Life: Achieving Optimal Health and Wellness through Ayurveda, Chinese Medicine, and Western Science*. Philadelphia: Da Capo Press, 2011.

Online Resources

Ali Cramer | alicramer.com | news, blogs, and links to supplies and information on upcoming trainings and events

The Ayurvedic Institute | ayurveda.com |

Banyan Botanicals | banyanbotanicals .com | Ayurvedic spices, herbs, tongue scrapers, neti pots, carrier oils, and information

Diaspora Co. | diasporaco.com | spices

Doterra for Essential Oils | doterra.com /US/en/site/alicramer

James Bae | baeacupuncture.com | acupuncture

Joyful Belly | joyfulbelly.com | Ayurvedic recipes and information

Kalustyan's | kalustyans.com | spices

Laughing Lotus | nyc.laughinglotus.com | Ayurvedic trainings

My Copper Cup | mycoppercup.co.uk | homemade copper cups and drinking bottles

National Eating Disorder Association | nationaleatingdisorders.org | eating disorder specialists

Pratima Skin Care| pratimaskincare.com | in-person spa treatments and incredible skin care

Robert Svoboda | youtube.com/channel /UCmcnwuSQls9-zdMbL2eenkA | short, informative videos on Ayurveda

Rod Stryker | youtube.com/user /RodStryker | yoga nidra videos

Scott Blossom | doctorblossom.com | Ayurvedic vaidya (doctor)

Somatheeram Ayurvedic Health Resort | somatheeram.org | Indian panchakarma center

Spotify | open.spotify.com /user/1240077361 | Ali's playlists

US Panchakarma | Center | https://www .ayurveda.com/

Victoria Koos | acupuncture-newyork.com | acupuncture

YogaAnytime | yogaanytime.com | online yoga classes

ACKNOWLEDGMENTS

Much gratitude to my Vata Mom, Doris, for her endless unquestioning support though all my unconventional choices. Much gratitude to my Pitta Dad, Allan, for his endless support and questioning of my choices throughout! Grateful for my Vata/Pitta brother, Peter, for questioning or not, depending on what was best for me. And, of course, Marty Cramer, for being so patient and keeping me company while I was holed up writing for hours.

Shout-out to my chosen family for their support and encouragement throughout this process—especially Sheri, Kenny, Deb, and Elian, who all told me to get on with it, listened to my first chapter, and gave me helpful feedback. To my student families at Laughing Lotus, WOOM Center, and around the world, thank you for your loyalty, receptivity, and devotion. Special thanks to Iana Velez of *NY YOGA + LIFE Magazine* and Joyce and Tracy for getting me to write again after a 20-year hiatus.

I am eternally grateful to my teachers, who have shared their wisdom, stories, and inspiration so generously: Dana Flynn, Jasmine Tarkeshi, Dr. Vasant Lad, Dr. Scott Blossom, Dr. Claudia Welch, Dr. Robert Svoboda, Maya Tiwari, Sarah Tomlinson, Morley Costello, and Nikki Costello. My prayer is to pass on even a fraction of your teachings in a way that is honorable, gentle, and, above all, loving.

Lastly, eternal thanks to Samantha Barbaro and the team at Althea Press, who made me actually sit down and write the book I kept thinking I would get to one day. One day became now. *Atha yoga anushasanam.*

In service,
Ali Cramer

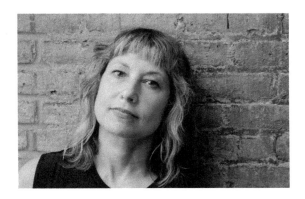

ABOUT THE AUTHOR

Ali Cramer is the director of the Ayurveda program at the Laughing Lotus yoga center in New York City. She has led trainings, workshops, and retreats both nationally and internationally since 2003. Her writing has been featured on many websites and in magazines, including *NY Yoga + Life* and *Mantra Wellness*. Stay in touch at alicramer.com.

CPSIA information can be obtained
at www.ICGtesting.com
Printed in the USA
LVHW052029180919
631492LV00004B/4/P